Adaptive Interaction and Dementia

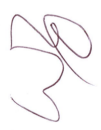

of related interest

Embracing Touch in Dementia Care
A Person-Centred Approach to Touch and Relationships
Luke Tanner
ISBN 978 1 78592 109 4
eISBN 978 1 78450 373 4

A Creative Toolkit for Communication in Dementia Care
Karrie Marshall
ISBN 978 1 84905 694 6
eISBN 978 1 78450 206 5

Positive Communication
Activities to Reduce Isolation and Improve the Wellbeing of Older Adults
Robin Dynes
ISBN 978 1 78592 181 0
eISBN 978 1 78450 449 6

Person-Centred Dementia Care, Second Edition
Making Services Better with the VIPS Framework
Dawn Brooker and Isabelle Latham
ISBN 978 1 84905 666 3
eISBN 978 1 78450 170 9

Adaptive Interaction and Dementia

How to Communicate without Speech

Maggie Ellis and **Arlene Astell**

Illustrations by **Suzanne Scott**

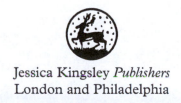

Jessica Kingsley *Publishers*
London and Philadelphia

First published in 2018
by Jessica Kingsley Publishers
73 Collier Street
London N1 9BE, UK
and
400 Market Street, Suite 400
Philadelphia, PA 19106, USA

www.jkp.com

Library of Congress Cataloging in Publication Data
Names: Ellis, Maggie (Psychologist), author. | Astell, Arlene, author.
Title: Adaptive interaction and dementia : how to communicate without speech
  / Maggie Ellis and Arlene Astell ; Illustrations by Suzanne Scott.
Description: London ; Philadelphia : Jessica Kingsley Publishers, 2018. |
  Includes bibliographical references and index.
Identifiers: LCCN 2017028861 | ISBN 9781785921971 (alk. paper)
Subjects: | MESH: Dementia | Aged | Communication Disorders | Nonverbal
  Communication
Classification: LCC RC524 | NLM WT 155 | DDC 616.8/31--
dc23 LC record available at https://lccn.loc.gov/2017028861

British Library Cataloguing in Publication Data
A CIP catalogue record for this book is available from the British Library

ISBN 978 1 78592 197 1
eISBN 978 1 78450 471 7

Printed and bound in Great Britain

We dedicate this book to our long-suffering husbands, Gordon and Paul, Arlene's youngest child, Izzie, and Maggie's dog, Jazzy, who have found for some time now that evenings and weekends are for book-writing. Thanks for your patience!

Acknowledgements

We would like to express gratitude to everyone who, over the years, has helped us in the development of Adaptive Interaction (AI). This includes, among many others, people with dementia, their family members and friends, formal caregivers, care home managers and academics. We are indebted and heartened by the commitment you have shown both to us and to Adaptive Interaction. Above all, we are grateful to you for putting your faith in an approach to communication that can elicit a range of feelings, for being willing to work through feelings of fear, uncertainty and self-consciousness to unearth joy, accomplishment and connection. Thank you.

We would also like to thank the illustrator of this book, Suzanne Scott. A recent chance meeting brought us together and we quickly realised we had met each other years ago. Good old serendipity! Suzanne has brought something very special to this book and we hope you love her illustrations as much as we do. Thanks Suzanne!

Contents

Preface

This book represents a culmination of our combined efforts over the last (almost) 16 years. Maggie came to work for Arlene as a research assistant, fresh out of an undergraduate degree in psychology. At that point, Arlene was relatively early on in her academic career and Maggie became her first PhD student. In that respect, you could say that we have 'grown up' together!

Adaptive Interaction is very special to us. We developed it with a shared passion for helping people with dementia who don't speak to connect with their families, friends and professional carers. It is an approach that we continue to research and one that we very much believe in. We strive to see it in use, at home and care facilities alike, and operate a tried and tested training programme that is available to anyone – from family members to care home managers to commissioners. We urge you to explore our website at www.astellis.co.uk where you will find details of how you can book a place on one of our courses. You will also find videos of Adaptive Interaction in use and hear the testimonies of those who use it.

One last point before we leave you to start your travels into Adaptive Interaction. You may notice that each chapter of this book contains a different song title. Why did we use this musical reference? That's easy. Songs represent little capsules of collaboration: collaboration between instruments, musicians, harmonies and rhythms. This is what Adaptive Interaction is all about – collaboration between people, their communication repertoires and the harmonies and rhythms that they 'play' together. Enjoy the music!

Maggie and Arlene

Chapter 1

Both Sides Now

Advanced Dementia from the Inside Out

What is this book about?

Adaptive Interaction and Dementia: How to Communicate without Speech is about losing your voice in a world dominated by words. Words are the glue of human existence. They shape our interactions in the world and connect us to other people. Every day we exchange millions of words through conversations, phone calls, emails, texts and so on. Just think for a moment how many words you have used today and the different ways you have used them. Aside from reading this book, how many texts or instant messages have you read or sent? How many emails or phone calls? How many chats and conversations?

Words enable us to be connected and this desire to be connected is universal. For instance, in 2015 there were over seven billion mobile phone subscriptions across the world (International Telecommunication Union (ITU), 2015) – as many as there were people on the planet in 2015. With these multiple channels of communication at our fingertips we can be in touch with other people all of the time. Not only is this big business, it is fundamental to human existence because humans are social beings. We live in social groups and spend our lives interacting and communicating with other people. We are continuously creating new ways of doing this. For instance, various 'textspeak' terms, including 'LOL', 'OMG', 'TMI' and 'BFF', entered the Oxford English Dictionary in 2011 (Oxford English Dictionary Online, 2011) and the Oxford Dictionaries Word of the Year 2015 was actually an emoji – 'face with tears of joy'. These confirm the importance of communication and connectedness in our lives and our constant desire to keep finding new ways to do it.

> **PAUSE FOR THOUGHT: THE MOBILE GENERATION**
>
> Most of us now carry phones or other devices with us all the time, which provide a sense of security and connectedness (Tennakoon and Taras, 2012). If you have a phone, have you ever lost it? How did you feel? Were you anxious? Annoyed? Upset? Did you think about all the things you need your phone for? What would you do if you didn't find it? What would be lost? If you found it again were you relieved? If you didn't see it again how did you cope? If you lost contents that you could not get back (e.g. photos, contacts) how did you feel?

I hope that you are now thinking about the multiple ways communication is embedded into our daily lives and how critical it is. Imagine then if your ability to interact with other people, your channels of communication, became impaired. If you became unable to hold conversations, to read, to write, to use a phone or to type. You would not be able to chat, speak on the phone, read or send emails, texts or instant messages. How would you express yourself? What would be the impact on your social interactions with your colleagues, your family and your friends? Would this affect your relationships? And how would it make you feel?

Many people living with dementia experience loss of communication skills like these. Their ability to speak and write may become impaired over time. Ultimately, people with dementia may no longer be able to use words at all. Typically, this will be after several years of living with dementia. If this happens individuals with dementia will also probably be reliant on other people for meeting other aspects of their daily needs and commonly they will be living in a care facility.

You can probably see by now that if you are no longer able to communicate with words, this has a profound impact on all aspects of your life. Everything shifts and starts to go on around you but without you. You become dependent on other people to include you and to keep you in the social world. Other people must make the effort to adapt their communication. But how can we communicate if we cannot use words?

This book addresses these communication issues as they relate to people with dementia who can no longer use words. Unlike people who are born unable to learn to speak, people with dementia gradually lose their capacity to speak or to understand speech, to write or to communicate with words in any way. This process of loss has a profound effect on all aspects of their lives: their ability to interact in the world, to exert control over what happens to them, to express their views, to stay connected with other people. The loss and changes people with dementia experience also affect their sense of self, their confidence in social interactions, and their relationships. They may withdraw from social situations through embarrassment or fear of saying or doing the wrong thing. By the point at which they are unable to use words, individuals with dementia may also be unable to walk or dress themselves, go to the toilet or eat independently.

In this book, we examine the specific challenges presented by dementia, particularly as these relate to communication and social interaction. However, this book is not about trying to 'fix' people who have dementia. While we explain the many challenges individuals with dementia face, we see that the solutions lie in enabling the people around them to make adaptations to the ways in which *they* communicate and to include the people with dementia as fellow human beings in the social world. Our first aim is to equip you as a reader with a good understanding of the challenges people with dementia experience in communicating and what that experience might be like. Our second aim is to provide you with an appreciation of the role individuals who interact with people who have dementia play in co-creating communication. These 'communication partners' are the other half of the equation when it comes to addressing the challenge of communicating without words. Our third aim is to provide you with an introduction to Adaptive Interaction – a means of communicating without words – and an understanding of how it can be integrated into the lives of people with dementia. We hope this book will open up a new way of understanding communication and of connecting with those who seem 'lost' to us.

What is dementia?

In the past 20 years, dementia has come to occupy the place that cancer once had. It is feared. It is poorly understood. And more and more people know someone who has been affected by it. In fact, dementia has existed and been recognised for as long as we have records. Greek philosophers believed that decline in mental abilities in old age was an inevitability if someone lived into their 60s or 70s. This notion that mental decline is an inevitable part of ageing was powerful and persisted until recent times. As such there was little investigation into possible causes of the cognitive decline that we now recognise as dementia until the 20th century. Before that time dementia was relatively rare, mainly because the biggest risk factor for developing dementia is age and lifespan was considerably lower than today. However, for most of the 20th century, dementia in later life was still considered a normal part of ageing.

The first case study of what became known as Alzheimer's disease (AD), presented by Alois Alzheimer in 1907, was of a 50-year-old woman (Alzheimer, 1907). She had distinctive changes in her brain and in her behaviour but at the time the case was regarded as an abnormal disease of middle age. It was not until the mid-1970s that neurologist Robert Katzman suggested there was a link between the changes in the brain he observed in people with AD and older people with dementia (Katzman, 1976). He and his colleagues argued that treating dementia as a normal part of ageing was preventing these people from being diagnosed with a disease. Katzman and Karasu (1975) proposed that rather than being rare and unusual, AD was probably among the top five causes of death among older people in the United States, but it was not being recorded on death certificates.

Since that time, the numbers of people living with dementia across the world have grown at a rapid pace, in part because people are living longer. In 2015, the number was estimated at 46.8 million, which is predicted to rise to 74.7 million by 2030 and 131.5 million by 2050 (Prince et al., 2015). What makes dementia particularly challenging is that it is not a single disorder. Alzheimer's disease is the most common cause of dementia, with current estimates suggesting it accounts for between 50 and 70 per cent of cases. Other types of dementia include vascular dementia, Lewy body dementia, frontotemporal dementia and several more, but the causes of these are even less well understood. Also, because many are relatively uncommon, they have been much less investigated than AD.

What we do know about all the dementias is that the changes that occur in the brain are irreversible and progressive and currently no drugs can halt or reverse the disease process. It is also well established that the changes in the brain often start many years before the person becomes aware that something is wrong. When they do so a clinical diagnosis is based on history of change and symptoms that can be assessed primarily through cognitive testing. In AD these include alterations in memory, thinking, and aspects of behaviour that interfere with an individual's ability to manage in everyday life. Frontotemporal dementias, which more commonly develop between 45 and 65 years of age, are particularly noted for changes in behaviour such as disinhibition, lack of empathy or emergence of rituals. There are also three subtypes of frontotemporal dementia – non-fluent aphasia, semantic dementia and logopenic aphasia (Onyike and Diehl-Schmid, 2013) – which are specifically characterised and diagnosed based on changes in speech and language. Although these dementia subtypes, collectively known as primary progressive aphasias, are uncommon, the impact of the language changes and the occurrence at a younger age are extremely difficult for people to deal with. For example, it has been shown that individuals with primary progressive aphasia commonly report symptoms of depression, including loss of interest and social withdrawal (Medina and Weintraub, 2007).

Because dementias are progressive, each person continues to experience changes in their cognitive functions and their behaviour, which increasingly interfere with their ability to carry out activities in everyday life such as shopping, cooking and driving. The changes people experience can be frightening, embarrassing and anxiety-provoking, and may lead them to withdraw from social situations. The reasons for this include not wanting to get things wrong and fear of negative evaluation by other people.

Let's consider your answers to these questions. If you are a reality television fan maybe you watch them because 'it's a laugh', or 'a bit of light relief', or 'so I can discuss it with my colleagues at work'. Maybe your reasons are for the human interest, because you care about what happens to the participants. If you do not watch reality shows it may be because these types of programme do not interest you. If you previously watched reality television but stopped perhaps you became bored with the format or no longer enjoy them. Or maybe you feel uncomfortable watching people being embarrassed or humiliated?

Our attitudes towards reality television provide interesting insights into the way the social world operates. Specifically, these programmes spotlight our reactions to other people's behaviour and the factors that influence them. These television shows encourage viewers to form opinions about the participants, both good and bad, based on what they say and do. By getting the viewer to develop an interest in what happens to the participants, the programme makers keep them coming back. Some people argue that reality television celebrates the worst aspects of human behaviour by laughing at the misfortune of others. There is evidence that participants are selected to maximise humiliation through 'gloating' at their weakness or failure (Mast, 2016). However, it has also been suggested that reality show viewers enjoy seeing other people in situations that they can empathise with (Hershman Shitrit and Cohen, 2016). Both the humiliation of other people and empathy with their situation are relevant for thinking about the changes people with dementia experience and how witnessing these might make us feel.

Some of these changes may frighten, embarrass or cause discomfort to other people who encounter them, including family, friends and wider society. This can lead to further exclusion from the social world as people avoid or minimise their contact with people who have dementia, in part to reduce their own discomfort. It has also been noted that some people respond by making fun of people with dementia and humiliating them by drawing attention to their problems or failings, perhaps as a means of distancing themselves from dementia or a reaction to their own inability to know how to respond. These 'personal detractors' (Kitwood, 1997) have been identified as one of the areas where training and education is most needed to improve the lives of people with dementia and those they interact with (see Chapter 2). Initiatives such as Dementia Friends (Alzheimer's Disease International, 2015) and Dementia-Friendly Communities (e.g. Wiersma and Denton, 2016) have sprung up in recent years to try to address some of these challenges in society at large. These activities aim to create educated populations who can support and enable people to live well with dementia. As most people live with dementia at home cared for by family and friends and with numbers predicted to keep rising, improving knowledge in the community is certainly to be welcomed.

However, some people who live with dementia do not have people to care for them at home. Others may have additional illnesses or other conditions that make it impossible for them to care for themselves. In these circumstances, people with dementia may find themselves being looked after by people they did not know before. This situation is challenging for people with dementia *and* the people who are employed to care for them. They are expected to develop a relationship at a time when the person with dementia may already be experiencing significant changes in their ability to communicate.

How does dementia impact communication?

Dementia affects communication in many ways. As we have seen above, there are three specific types of dementia that primarily affect speech and language. People living with other dementias can also have problems finding words and answering simple questions. They may repeat what is said to them. As with most aspects of dementia, the changes in speech and communication have been most investigated in AD, the most common cause of dementia. People with AD find it increasingly difficult to keep hold of information during a conversation. Consequently, their speech may often seem repetitive and difficult to follow and they make more speech errors (Bayles and Tomoeda, 1993). Over time people with AD take shorter conversational turns with longer pauses between these turns and may change topic without warning. These alterations affect the flow of conversation, making it difficult for a person they are interacting with to know when to speak.

21

In addition, communication partners of people with AD report an increase in disjointed speech and discussion of topics that the partner judges 'meaningless' (Bayles and Tomoeda, 1991). These changes may result in interactions that are both demanding and dissatisfying, particularly to communication partners who may feel their contributions are being marginalised (Astell et al., 2005). It has been suggested that communication partners interpret repetition by people with AD either as the person with dementia not listening to them, or being deliberately difficult. Both interpretations may contribute to subsequent strain and tension in their relationships (Almberg, Grafström and Winblad, 1997).

Taken together it is clear that dementia of all types has a global impact on speech and communication as the illness progresses, which creates problems for people with a diagnosis and their potential communication partners. Professional staff and family members are faced with the challenge of making themselves understood in the face of their own decreasing ability to understand those they are interacting with (Bayles and Tomoeda, 1991). This assault on the ability to communicate may be *the* most frustrating and upsetting impact of dementia both for people with dementia and those they interact with (Azuma and Bayles, 1997). Kate Swaffer, an Australian woman living with semantic dementia since 2008, posted the following blog in 2013:

Talking eventually becomes an embarrassment or humil-iation for a person with dementia... The difficulty with being embarrassed about talking is it tends to isolate [people with dementia] even more. It can feel easier to let the phone ring out, than make a fool of myself. Maybe this is why people with dementia start to give up communicating. Perhaps it is not only the difficulty we have with things like word finding, but also the humiliation of having to listen to ourselves stumble and jumble with our words? Of course, our family and friends don't mind, but how we feel about these changes must surely colour the way we respond to the symptoms of dementia? Is it simply easier to say nothing, than to humiliate ourselves?

As discussed above, humiliation is a powerful social influence and Kate's words sum up very well the experiences of many people with dementia. They seek to avoid feeling humiliated and so reduce communication and situations when they could interact with others. Arguably this is a normal human response as we generally seek to avoid feeling humiliated.

People who have dementia who can no longer use words find themselves in a different position. It is difficult to see how they can act on their environment to diminish humiliation. This is not just because they do not have words but because of the other changes they have probably experienced, such as inability to walk or get out of bed. As such they rely on other people to enable them to act in the world and to reduce the occurrence of situations where they may experience humiliation. Even though people may no longer be able to use words this does not mean the end of communication.

Early in our research we established that the urge to communicate is retained even if words are not (Ellis and Astell, 2004). This is indicated in multiple ways through nonverbal means including sounds, movements, eye gaze and other responses to people in their environment. What is required is for potential communication partners to recognise and respond to these communication bids from people with dementia who can no longer use words.

Communication is a two-way thing

When you think about it, it is obvious that communication is a two-way thing. We do not communicate alone. Our communications are with other people. Be it face to face or remotely, we interact with other people.

PAUSE FOR THOUGHT: CONVEYING MESSAGES

Think about the last time you phoned someone or sent an email or text or instant message. What were you trying to convey? Did you expect a response or reaction? Did you receive the response you wanted? Did it matter to you how the person responded?

Now think about the person you communicated with. Was it a significant other or a friend or a parent or a child or a colleague or your boss? Think again about what you were trying to convey. What sort of reaction or response were you hoping for? Did you receive the response that you wanted? If you did, how did you feel? If you did not receive the response you hoped for, how did you feel?

This activity reminds us of the importance of other people in communication. When we encounter someone who has a communication difficulty it is up to us to adjust and modify our behaviour to encourage communication. 'Conversational repair' refers to the actions of parties in a conversation to resolve misunderstandings or mis-hearings that occur. The process of conversational repair is 'collaborative, generally formulaic, and includes problematic utterance(s), the signal of a problem, and the repair of the problem' (Orange, Lubinksi and Higginbotham, 1996, p. 882). People with AD can repair conversational misunderstandings, but over time the percentage of conversation that involves repair increases, placing greater demands on their conversation partner (Orange et al., 1996).

As conversational repair is collaborative, the role of the partner is crucial. In the Orange et al. study (1996), conversation partners were family members who had long knowledge and experience of conversations with the individuals with dementia, and arguably more vested interest in keeping them going.

Staff in care settings must get to know people with impaired communication and provide opportunities for meaningful social interaction and participation. In a study of conversations in care homes, Baker et al. (2015) identified three types of conversations. The first type was defined by staff initiating topics and doing most of the talking. In the second type of conversation, the amount of conversation was more even and people with dementia initiated some topics. In the third conversation type, people with dementia spoke the most with staff supporting them. Analysis of the different conversation types identified helpful strategies that staff used to keep their partners with dementia engaged, such as repeating back what they said. The authors also highlighted staff behaviours that were unhelpful, such as not fully paying attention and not giving enough time to their partner to speak.

Uncovering and maximising the communication skills that people with dementia retain is crucial for improving their lives (Kitwood, 1997). Predictably, this becomes more difficult to accomplish as communication changes and people lose the ability to use words. The 'person-centred approach' (Brooker, 2003; Kitwood, 1997) provides a framework for identifying retained communication skills and exploration of how these can be maximised to support meaningful interactions between people with dementia and caregivers. The focus is on identifying and meeting the needs of the person, and aims to enhance wellbeing by improving relationships and communication between people with dementia, their families and professional caregivers. 'Person-centredness' is achieved when people interacting with the individual focus more on them as a fellow human being than on the illness.

In her 2006 book, Dawn Brooker proposed 'VIPS' as the four main elements that should be addressed in person-centred care: Valuing people with dementia and their caregivers (V); regarding people with dementia as Individuals (I); looking at the world from the Perspective of people with dementia (P); and creating a positive Social environment to allow the person with dementia to experience relative wellbeing (S). Any strategy to facilitate communication between people with dementia and their caregivers or to maintain a sense of self in people with dementia should, in theory, contain these essentials. In so doing, the onus is placed very much on the caregiver or communication partner to ensure that these elements are fully addressed. The relationship between people with dementia, their family members and professional caregivers (the dementia care triad) is critical for improving wellbeing (Woods, Keady and Seddon, 2007). This highlights the need to explore the nature and quality of relationships between members of the care triad as well as the impact of dementia on individuals with a diagnosis. We take a collaborative approach to addressing how communication partners can facilitate people with dementia who can no longer use words to interact and stay in the social world.

What is Adaptive Interaction?

This book tells the story of Adaptive Interaction – a means of communicating without words – which we developed to address the communication gap when people with dementia can no longer use words. We are sharing our experience as a resource for anyone interacting with individuals who have dementia and can no longer speak. Adaptive Interaction grew out of Intensive Interaction (II) (Nind and Hewett, 1994), an established approach well known in the fields of intellectual disability and autism spectrum disorders (ASD). Many years ago, we were fortunate to receive training in II from the amazing Phoebe Caldwell. Phoebe came to stay with us and together we practised the basics of II. This experience profoundly influenced our thinking and our approach to using nonverbal communication with people with dementia who can no longer use words and we are eternally grateful to Phoebe for sharing her wisdom and expertise with us and for continuing to inspire.

Phoebe taught us the importance of 'learning the language of the individual'. The term 'language' might seem odd when we think about communicating without words. But language is so much more than words. We come into the world equipped to connect with other human beings. Babies are born with a set of behaviours – the so-called 'fundamentals of communication' – designed to trigger a response from parents and caregivers. Initially, this is to ensure survival of the infant. It is also the basis for developing speech.

The fundamentals of communication include shared attention, eye gaze, sounds, movement and imitation. Babies are programmed to make eye contact and imitate simple actions (such as poking their tongues out) right from birth (Meltzoff and Moore, 1983). As speech starts to develop, these nonverbal means of communication become less relied on, but they do not go away. Shrugs, hugs, tears and smiles are all integral to our everyday communication. They accentuate, reinforce and frequently replace words. And if speech and other means of using words do disappear, as experienced by many people with dementia, these fundamentals of communication remain.

To learn the language of a person with dementia who cannot use words we focus on these fundamentals of communication. We study their eye gaze, facial expressions, sounds and movements. From this we develop a profile of each person's communication repertoire. Some individuals' repertoires are dominated by sounds, others by eye gaze and yet others by very subtle movements. What we have learnt is that everyone has their own individual repertoire and that it is possible to identify it and use this 'language' to make connections with individuals with dementia who can no longer use words. In so doing, we help to keep people with advanced dementia in the social world.

Having learnt their language, we look for communicative behaviours to home in on and re-establish a connection. We also try initiating connections using elements of their own repertoires, such as sounds or movements, but we always allow the individual to lead. Our experience has taught us to be open minded about each interaction, not to expect to pick up where we left off, and ready to adapt to each person and each encounter. Hence, Adaptive Interaction was born.

To illustrate our approach, we will use the stories of Chrissie, Eleanor and Bert, imaginary residents of the fictional Roseford Care Home, who each have a different and distinct communication repertoire. These stories are composites drawn from multiple individuals we have had the joy and pleasure of getting to know using Adaptive Interaction. We have chosen these three stories to highlight the huge variability between people who are living with dementia and who can no longer use words. We also want to ensure that the personhood of every single individual living with dementia is recognised and valued.

CHRISSIE

Chrissie is 78 years old and has been resident in Roseford Care Home for three years. She worked in a mill for most of her working life and enjoyed the company of the many friends she made there. A very outgoing and funny woman, Chrissie had a 'wicked' sense of humour and would often play practical jokes on her colleagues and family members. She loved to sing and would take every chance she could to get a sing-song going at parties and get-togethers. Her friends described her as the life and soul of the party and she never turned down a chance to gather with friends and family. She and her husband Phil had four children and were happily married for 43 years until Phil died suddenly of a massive stroke.

Chrissie's family found out very quickly when Phil died just how much he had been doing for Chrissie behind the scenes. They had previously noticed that Chrissie was having some, what they thought to be, minor memory problems but they put that down to her 'getting older'. After Phil died she was quickly diagnosed with dementia after going outside in her nightdress early in the morning. She was found, outside the university building where her daughter Jean worked, at 6 a.m. The police were called and Chrissie became a resident at Roseford soon after.

ELEANOR

Eleanor is 66 years old and has been living in Roseford Care Home for seven years. Eleanor was diagnosed with a type of early onset dementia when she was 55 years old. Eleanor has one daughter, Angie, with whom she is very close. She is also married to Mike – a very supportive man who is clearly devoted to her and her wellbeing. He describes himself as her husband, not her 'carer', and is quick to correct anyone who fails to make this distinction. Eleanor is extremely fortunate in terms of her family's commitment to her as she has regular visits from her family.

Eleanor's early dementia became apparent when she started to make mistakes at work and the usually self-confident nurse became more and more withdrawn and unsure. She would typically attempt to cover up her mistakes with a joke and a laugh – never for a minute acknowledging that anything was wrong. At other times, Eleanor would blame her colleagues for her mistakes in a desperate attempt to save face. This upset her work mates and they began to detach themselves from her whenever possible.

Eleanor started avoiding nights out with work colleagues and stopped gathering with them at coffee breaks. She was embarrassed by what was happening to her and wanted to maintain her status and friendships but finally it became too much to manage. The situation came to a head when Eleanor's daughter returned from her gap year and noticed a marked change in her mum's demeanour. Angie made an appointment for her mum with the GP and accompanied her to the meeting. Not long after this, Eleanor was diagnosed with early onset dementia and gave up work.

BERT

Bert is 85 years old and has been living in Roseford Care Home for the past five years. He is a very quiet and gentle man who spent his working life as a ranger at a local wildlife park. He retired at 65 years of age and enjoyed a peaceful and relatively solitary existence until he was 78. Before moving to Roseford, Bert was somewhat of a loner and spent most of his time walking in the woods with his dog, Isla. Although outwardly friendly, he had no close friends or family and never married or had a partner. Bert's passion in life was nature and as such the outdoor life of a park ranger suited him. He tended to avoid large groups, preferring instead to keep himself to himself.

Bert was diagnosed with dementia when he was 79. This was after his neighbours became concerned when he started walking Isla in the middle of the night. Some nights the dog returned home but Bert was still out. One night, Bert's neighbour Betty found Isla, still in her collar and lead, barking outside her companion's door at 4 a.m. She took the dog indoors and her husband Frank went out to look for Bert. Frank found Bert in the woods near his home. He was physically well but very confused, cold and upset. That evening's events prompted Betty and Frank to keep an eye on Bert from thereon in. They would visit him every day and he would come over to their house on Sundays for dinner. Bert seemed to enjoy their company despite his retiring nature and always looked genuinely pleased to see them. It seemed to Betty and Frank that all Bert needed was someone to make the first move and show an interest in him.

Bert's behaviour changed significantly over the course of the following year as Betty and Frank noticed that he was losing weight and becoming unsteady on his feet. Frank started to walk Isla to help Bert out but sometimes Bert would forget who his neighbour was when he came to the door. Eventually Bert refused to open the door to his neighbours and they would hear Isla barking and howling in distress. Frank and Betty called Social Services as they were so concerned about Bert and Isla's welfare. He was assessed, diagnosed with dementia and quickly moved to Roseford as he was deemed no longer able to care for himself or for his dog. Betty and Frank adopted Isla and still take her to visit him at the care home to this day.

Communicating without words

In the following chapters, we get to know Chrissie, Eleanor and Bert better and learn how dementia has caused each of them to slip out of the social world in different ways. We will also meet their family and friends and care staff who are seeking to connect and interact with them. Each one is paired with a communication partner – respectively Stacey, James and Betty – who you will also follow. We will examine how Adaptive Interaction enables their communication partners to identify their individual communication repertoires, learn their language and develop ways of communicating without words. In Chapter 2 we find out more about Eleanor, Bert and Chrissie to gain an understanding of dementia from the inside out. We also examine the role of the interaction partner in co-creating the social world of people with dementia who can no longer use words. In Chapter 3 we introduce the concept of collaborative communication, a model of human interaction that emphasises the role of both partners in communication, and consider how this could enable Eleanor, Bert and Chrissie to continue as social participants. Chapter 4 describes Adaptive Interaction and explores in detail the processes involved in learning the language of individuals with dementia who can no longer use words to elicit their communication repertoires. Chapters 5, 6 and 7 each focus on one person, following them and their communication partner as they learn to use Adaptive Interaction. Chapter 5 considers Chrissie's situation and the challenges of interacting with someone who makes lots of sounds. Chapter 6 examines Eleanor's situation and the communicative nature of behaviour. Chapter 7 focuses on Bert's story and looks at communication with someone who makes no sounds at all.

Chapter 2

We've Only Just Begun
Learning the Language of Dementia

In this chapter, you will learn more about Chrissie, Eleanor and Bert, and some of the challenges faced by individuals like them who are living with dementia and who cannot speak. You will also find out more about the challenges faced by the people who try to interact with them. This includes examining the importance we attach to the ability to speak in social interactions and the impact that speech loss has on both people with dementia and their interaction partners.

The impact of dementia on relationships
BERT

Bert, who was previously an active although solitary man, is no longer able to walk and is quite removed from the social activity in Roseford. He no longer speaks and seems to be completely unaware that he has company when his neighbours Frank and Betty, and his dog Isla, come to visit. He does not make eye contact with them and never utters a sound. He mostly spends his days sleeping and when he is awake, he seems to stare into space. Frank and Betty find it very upsetting to see

Bert like this and start to visit him less and less as they are at a loss how to communicate with him.

Many difficulties that occur between people with dementia and those who care for them arise directly from the cognitive changes that characterise dementia. For example, when people first develop dementia they may experience memory and planning problems, which mean they need help to carry out everyday tasks. This can take the form of someone checking that activities have been completed and that individuals with dementia are keeping on top of their work or daily activities. Over time people may need more reminding, including where they are, what day it is, what time it is and what they were just doing, and so on. The constant need for monitoring and reassurance undoubtedly weighs heavily both on people with dementia and the people who interact with them. As you might expect, these difficulties can impact hugely on their relationships. For families, this can put a strain on maintaining existing relationships. For care staff, they must develop relationships with people who have already experienced significant cognitive loss and changes to their ability to communicate effectively.

As time passes and an individual's need for assistance grows, there is often a narrowing of focus from caregivers. Checking that tasks are carried out commonly transforms into close supervision of all steps of a task such as cooking or shopping. With further cognitive decline, there is increased need for direct input from caregivers in all aspects of daily life. For example, as an individual becomes less able to wash, to eat without assistance, to walk and so on, caregivers find that more and more of the time spent together is filled with these tasks. In addition, the increasing physical care that people with dementia require, such as help with going to the toilet and bathing, may be embarrassing for their partners or children. It is also physically demanding, which may contribute to caregivers having less energy to spend on social interactions.

BETTY

Betty still visits Bert with Frank and Isla but finds the visits difficult as he seems so disconnected. They thought that Isla would be a spark for Bert but he no longer reacts to his dog and Betty and Frank end up sitting in awkward silence or speaking to each other and hoping in vain something will capture Bert's attention. This once active, busy man who spent hours every day out walking in the countryside he loved is now a shell of his former self. Betty is upset to see him this way and struggles to know how best to interact with him, but she does not want to give up as he has no one else. However, she is finding it harder and harder to go to Roseford as it makes her feel so sad and uncomfortable.

In addition to the reactions of others, people with dementia may experience difficulties interpreting social situations from quite an early stage. Social cognition describes the relationship between social behaviour and the underlying cognitive processes that support it. Unsurprisingly, people who have cognitive impairments also have difficulties reading cues in social situations. Rapid automatic processing of the basic, universal emotions is a fundamental component of social communication that we are born with (Batty and Taylor, 2003). The face and body provide immediate nonverbal indicators of other people's internal states, sending powerful cues as to how they are feeling. Thus, difficulty picking up on social cues could lead to misunderstanding and inappropriate behaviour.

However, it appears that the problems faced by people with dementia are not so much to do with detecting emotion in others, but rather with interpreting the complex information contained in social situations. For instance, they retain the ability to recognise the basic emotions from photographs of faces (Astell, Ellis and Hockey, 2004). However, when faced with interpreting complex social scenes containing one or more people, they are much less likely to make inferences about the feelings and motivations of characters, sticking instead to concrete descriptions of items in the scenes (Astell et al., 2004). This has practical implications for everyday interactions with friends and family members and is another source of misunderstanding and hurt feelings that arise in the relationships of people with dementia.

Family relationships

One common source of problems in families is that people with dementia may fail to recognise family members and significant people, events and places, either in life or in photographs. Relatives often feel hurt and rejected if their family member with dementia fails to recognise them or significant family events such as weddings or birthday parties. This is likely because photographs have emotional significance for family members and they expect them to have the same resonances for people with dementia, or that the emotional 'connectedness' will make them more memorable (Astell et al., 2010). However, this fails to take into account the changes in the brain experienced by people with dementia that make it difficult for them to make and retain new memories. Therefore people, places and events they encountered after their brain started to lose neurons and connections are unlikely to be remembered explicitly, either because they have not laid down memories of these recent events or they cannot access them (Shenk, 2001). However, the failure to recognise the people or places may suggest to family members that they are not important to the people with dementia, which can influence their views of the individual.

Orange and Purves (1996) noted that the nature of relationships can influence the quality of interactions between people with dementia and their communication partners. Family caregivers find themselves in particularly challenging circumstances, as they are typically provided with very little information about the impact of dementia and little or no training in how to care for someone with the illness (Hepburn et al., 2001). Family caregivers find this very difficult and may experience significant stress (Zarit and Edwards, 2008). Where the caregiver is a husband or wife, the transition from partnership to caregiving and dependency is typically very difficult to deal with. For many couples this change occurs after they have spent a lifetime together and thus the caring partner often feels that they have lost the person they have shared their life with. The impact of this shift is influenced by the quality of the pre-care relationship, while the amount of assistance needed by the person with dementia affects the caregiver's perceptions of the current state of the relationship (Quinn, Clare and Woods, 2009).

Crucially, family members may be unaware that their own behaviour has an impact on the person they care for (Kitwood, 1990). Therefore, many of the symptoms of dementia are misinterpreted and may be unintentionally exacerbated by family members (Kitwood, 1997). For example, it may appear that the personality of a person with dementia has changed, as their behaviour and reactions to people and situations is different from before they developed dementia. This interpretation of personality change by family members is cited as one of the most prevalent and distressing symptoms to deal with (Chatterjee et al., 1992). Indeed, even small changes in character or increases in so-called problematic behaviour, such as forgetting, uncharacteristic aggressive reactions or constant walking, can cause family members to feel resentment towards their relatives with dementia. When care recipients have greater needs for assistance, especially in marital relationships, this can manifest in potentially harmful caregiver behaviours such as 'screaming and yelling, insulting or swearing, threatening to send to a nursing home, and withholding food' (Beach et al., 2005, p. 255). Clearly such reactions are not good for anyone.

In an exploration of 'compassion fatigue' among family caregivers, Day and Anderson (2011) found evidence of hopelessness, helplessness, emotional disengagement and apathy, four indicators commonly found in health care professionals who are experiencing difficulties in their work. Emotional disengagement, where 'family members of a person with dementia…have feelings of disgust, embarrassment, and decreased involvement' leads to compassion fatigue and withdrawal from the individual with dementia (Day and Anderson, 2011, p. 6). This results in people with dementia being excluded from the social world at a time when they are most in need of other people to keep them in it.

Research addressing the impact of dementia on family relationships suggests that from the outset there should be discussion and proactive meaning making about the diagnosis of dementia in the family. For couples, Robinson, Clare and Evans (2005) proposed that they 'may be supported by helping them to create a joint construction that enables them to make sense of their situation, find ways of adjusting to the changes experienced in their roles and identity, and manage the losses they face in the early stages of dementia' (p. 337). Despite this good advice, there has been little systematic effort to support and encourage families to participate in such positive activities and thus the experiences of individual families living with dementia has changed little, even though awareness and publicity about dementia has been growing at an extraordinary pace over the last ten years.

Relationships with formal caregivers

More research has been conducted into relationships between formal caregivers and people with dementia than family caregivers. Poor attitudes towards people with dementia have long been associated with high 'burnout' in care staff (Aström et al., 1991; Berg, Hansson and Hallberg, 1994). Poor motivation and training among staff in residential care settings can lead to reduced levels of staff–resident interactions as staff feel unable and/or unsupported to communicate with people with dementia (Burgio et al., 1990; Carstensen, Fisher and Malloy, 1995). As with family caregivers, lack of knowledge in these areas can often lead to a misinterpretation of the communication attempts of people with dementia and, therefore, less effort by care staff to interact. This lack of social contact is undoubtedly detrimental to both individuals with dementia and care staff, and highlights the importance of maximising the potential for interaction in the social environment.

Caregiver attitudes and behaviour can be significantly improved by education about the cognitive and social impact of dementia and the existence of significantly spared abilities in those with a diagnosis (Berg et al., 1994; Chappell and Novak, 1992). Providing information in these areas improves how formal caregivers regard people with dementia, their relationships with those they care for and their own levels of job satisfaction (Berg et al., 1994; Chappell and Novak, 1992; Constable and Russell, 1986). Education is also needed to challenge negative expectations caregivers bring to the communication environment. While family caregivers bring their memories and prior relationships to the caregiving situation, there is evidence that professional caregivers have both negative and low expectations about the abilities of people with dementia. This is at the root of the 'malignant social psychology' in dementia care identified by Kitwood (1990; see the section 'Malignant social psychology' below). Staff attitudes towards the severity of dementia can also have a knock-on effect on staff–resident communication (Burgio et al., 1990; Carstensen et al., 1995). For example, it has been reported that nursing aides who use facilitative conversation strategies such as providing reminders, cues and encouragements, have more conversations with residents with early dementia than those at more advanced stages (Dijkstra et al., 2002). However, it is people at the later stages of the illness who are in the greatest need of help to communicate (Dijkstra et al., 2002).

Changes in behaviour

ELEANOR

A previously gregarious nurse with many friends, 11 years after her diagnosis of early onset dementia, Eleanor no longer speaks and appears unable to communicate at all. She has a steely look in her eye, which she seems to reserve for those people she does not like very much. However, the object of this glare can change. One day it might be the doctor, the next day the cleaner or a visiting neighbour – no-one can be sure when she might turn her unsettling gaze on them. The care staff tend to avoid Eleanor if they can as they find her behaviour unpredictable and hostile, especially during personal care, when she can become very upset. At these times, she can hit out and push them away when they come to assist her to go to the toilet or have a shower. Neither the care staff nor her family have any idea why this might be and care staff typically dread these types of activities as they know that Eleanor will become extremely distressed.

Approximately half of people with dementia are reported by caregivers to experience changes in their behaviour or for new behaviours to emerge, such as agitation, anxiety, mood or sleep disturbance (Stoppe, Brandt and Staedt, 1999). These changes have been commonly termed 'challenging behaviour' as they present a challenge to caregivers, both formal and informal. Over time this phrase has become regarded as critical of people with dementia, resulting in attempts to replace it with terms such as 'responsive behaviours' (Gutmanis et al., 2015) or behavioural and psychological symptoms of dementia (BPSD) (Feast et al., 2016). In all cases the labelling of this behaviour locates the problem onto the individual with dementia, for instance classifying it as a 'symptom' of dementia, and something that must be managed. This location of the problem on the individuals with dementia influences most of the efforts to address these difficulties.

Behavioural changes, along with incontinence, have long been cited as the most common reasons for care at home to break down (O'Donnell et al., 1992) and a recent review identified two main reasons that family carers identified behaviour as challenging (Feast et al., 2016). The first was associated with the changes in their communication and relationships, leaving the caregiver feeling 'bereft'. Second was caregiver feelings of 'transgression of social norms' arising from a lack of understanding of the changes in behaviour a person with dementia can experience. The 'sense of a declining relationship' and 'belief that their relative had lost, or would inevitably lose, their identity to dementia' (p. 429) were major determinants of family caregivers describing their relative's behaviour as challenging.

In formal care settings, the behaviour of people with dementia is also a significant focus of attention. In a survey of 326 staff working in 14 care homes in England, Moniz-Cook, Woods and Gardiner (2000) found that staff anxiety, perceived or actual support from a supervisor, and 'the potential to relate to residents as individuals' (p. 48) were the main predictors of staff identifying resident behaviour as challenging. Like family caregivers, many care staff find it stressful to deal with behaviour they deem challenging (Hazelhof et al., 2016). In their recent concept analysis, Hazelhof et al. (2016, p. 507) identified a wide range of factors relating, first, to residents (described as 'physical and verbal aggression, conflicts, excessive demands, being unresponsive') and, second, to nursing staff ('age, experience, tenure, nursing level and training'), that influence staff stress. Interventions to reduce the frequency of behaviour that staff find challenging and improving communication between staff at all levels may be helpful for enabling staff to better deal with such occurrences (Koder, Hunt and Davison, 2014).

JAMES

James is one of the younger staff at Roseford who has only been working there for about six months. When he first started working on the unit where Eleanor lives, he shadowed other, more experienced members of staff. Whenever they went into Eleanor's room they warned him to beware of getting too close to her as she could hit out unexpectedly. They also told him about her icy glare and how she made them feel uncomfortable. As he spends more time with Eleanor and takes on more responsibility for her care, James begins to feel that she is missing out on social interaction as the only times people really interacted with her is during personal care, which they try to complete as quickly as possible. He would like to do more for Eleanor but does not know how to do things differently.

It has been suggested that the reason for a behaviour being labelled as 'challenging' is often the perception of home carers or care staff, and the discomfort, uncertainty or fear caused by the behaviour, as opposed to the actual behaviour itself (Bird et al., 2002). However, actions such as shouting, following a caregiver or weeping can be argued to be serving a communication function, indicating to caregivers that a person with dementia is distressed, or some other need, wish or desire to communicate

(Stokes, 2000). Constant walking or picking things up can indicate boredom or lack of stimulation. Similarly, a person asking to go home or stating that their mother is waiting for them may be trying to reduce their own anxiety, aroused from being in what is, to them, an unfamiliar surrounding, by seeking a place of familiarity and comfort. Recognising the communicative behaviour and addressing the unmet needs of people with dementia can promote their autonomy and enhance the provision of dignified care from nursing staff (Smith and Buckwalter, 2005).

Malignant social psychology

Kitwood (1997) coined the term 'malignant social psychology' to describe what he saw as the prevalent and pervasive attitude towards people with dementia. This phenomenon arises from the interaction between the neurological impairments experienced by people with dementia and the negative attitudes of those around them. It is important to point out that in using the term 'malignant' Kitwood (1997) was not referring to any ill intent of caregivers towards people with dementia. Rather, malignancy in this context referred to the nature of our 'cultural inheritance' (Kitwood, 1997, p. 46). In other words, our culture has historically had a negative approach to individuals with neurological or cognitive impairments. The resulting malignant social psychology is known to have a significant negative impact on the wellbeing of people with dementia and may even hasten further cognitive decline. As we saw in Chapter 1, humiliation occurs when we experience being 'unjustly degraded, ridiculed or put-down – in particular, our identity has been demeaned or devalued' (Hartling and Luccheta, 1999). This is the consequence of the way one or more other people behave towards us. Humiliating acts are behaviours that 'lower a person's or group's dignity or self-esteem, with the perpetrator often deriving a sense of self-satisfaction from it by feeling *above* [original italics] the other' (Mast, 2016, p. 2185).

PAUSE FOR THOUGHT: EMBARRASSMENT

We have all had the experience of doing something embarrassing in front of family, friends, colleagues or strangers. This could be coming out of the toilet with paper trailing behind you, discovering you have not fastened an article of clothing or breaking wind in a public place. Take a moment to think of an embarrassing situation you have been in. How did you feel? How did you deal with the situation?

How we feel depends a lot on the reaction of other people. Humans have a desire to fit in or belong to social groups and so we constantly look at what other people think of us. Thinking back to your own experience, can you recall who else was there and how they reacted? Did they tease you or look shocked? Did they say anything to you about what happened? If so, was it consoling or accusing? How did *their* reaction make you feel?

How you dealt with the situation will have been partly influenced by the reactions of these other people. Typically, we adopt one of two strategies for dealing with embarrassing situations – avoidance or confrontation. Avoidance speaks for itself in pretending that the bad or awkward thing did not happen. Confrontation means you directly address the embarrassing incident, either by making a joke or, depending on the situation, apologising. What did you do in the situation you are recalling?

Embarrassment is common among caregivers of people with dementia and has been found to be associated with depression (Springate and Tremont, 2014). It is not hard to see that avoidance could be adopted by caregivers as a response to their embarrassment, which is often accompanied by frustration.

The ways caregivers respond to the behaviour of people with dementia are largely dependent on their perceptions of whether those with a diagnosis can exert control over their behaviour (Paton et al., 2004). Indeed, family members have reported that they consider that most of the 'symptoms' of dementia they witness are under the control of those they care for. In short, family caregivers often felt that many of the behaviours they found problematic were premeditated and deliberate (Paton et al., 2004). Due to this belief, caregivers may engage in behaviour towards the person they care for that in some way detracts from the personhood of the individual with dementia. These negative caregiver behaviours are known as 'personal detractors' (Kitwood, 1990). These include infantilisation, marginalisation or even completely ignoring people with dementia. The following table describes the 17 'personal detractors' Kitwood identified.

Table 2.1 Personal detractors described by Kitwood (1990)

Category	Description	Example
Treachery	Using forms of deception to distract or manipulate a person, or force them into compliance.	Telling Mary that her daughter will be here soon to take her home, when in fact she no longer lives at home and her daughter lives on the other side of the world.
Disempowerment	Not allowing a person to use the abilities that they do have; failing to help them to complete actions that they have initiated.	Taking John's cutlery away from him and 'feeding' him when you think he is taking 'too long'.
Infantilisation	Treating a person very patronisingly (or 'matronisingly') as an insensitive parent might treat a very young child.	Telling Michael that he is being 'very naughty' when he swears at another resident.
Intimidation	Inducing fear in a person, through threats or physical power.	Telling Isobel that you will 'make' her sit still if she doesn't stop walking around the home.
Labelling	Using a category such as dementia or 'organic mental disorder' as the main basis for interacting with a person and for explaining their behaviour.	Talking about Sandra and Tracey as 'demented patients'.

Category	Description	Example
Stigmatisation	Treating a person as if they were a diseased object, an alien or an outcast.	Closing the door on Graham when he has experienced incontinence.
Outpacing	Providing information, presenting choices, etc., at a rate too fast for a person to understand; putting them under pressure to do things more rapidly than they can bear.	Telling Theresa to 'hurry up' when she is getting undressed for her shower.
Invalidation	Failing to acknowledge the subjective reality of a person's experience and, especially, what they are feeling.	Telling Morris not to be 'silly' when he is upset and asks to see his mum.
Banishment	Sending a person away, or excluding them – physically or psychologically.	Taking Bob to his room and closing the door because he is 'wailing'.
Objectification	Treating a person as if they were a lump of dead matter: to be pushed, lifted, filled, pumped or drained, without proper reference to the fact that they are sentient beings.	Talking and laughing with a colleague about something unrelated when washing and dressing Shona.
Ignoring	Carrying on (in conversation or action) in the presence of a person as if they were not there.	Chatting to your colleague while Sally is asking to go to the toilet.
Imposition	Forcing a person to do something, overriding desire or denying the possibility of choice on their part.	Spooning rice pudding into Imogen's mouth when she has already said she didn't want any.
Withholding	Refusing to give asked-for attention, or to meet an evident need.	Watching the news on TV and telling Arthur he'll just have to wait when he says he's hungry.
Accusation	Blaming a person for actions or failures of action that arise from their lack of ability, or their misunderstanding of the situation.	Sending Theresa out of the room when the art therapist is in because she 'doesn't concentrate'.
Disruption	Intruding suddenly or disturbingly upon a person's action or reflection; crudely breaking their frame of reference.	Putting a glass of juice into Tom's hand while he is flicking through a newspaper.
Mockery	Making fun of a person's 'strange' actions or remarks; teasing, humiliating, making jokes at their expense.	Laughing at Gina with colleagues because she is pouring sugar instead of milk into her teacup.
Disparagement	Telling a person that they are incompetent, useless, worthless, etc., giving them messages that are damaging to their self-esteem.	Laughing and telling Michael that he is 'rubbish' when he tries to remember how to play a tune on the piano.

Although it is nearly 30 years since Kitwood presented the concept of malignant social psychology and despite the enshrinement of person-centredness as the centrepiece of dementia care, these responses to people with dementia persist. In large part this is due to lack of education and training about dementia, especially for family caregivers who are largely left to figure out for themselves how to interact and respond to their relative with dementia. But this also happens in dementia care services where the focus is on completing tasks rather than interacting and spending time with people with dementia. As such, it is easier if they sit quietly and do not make demands on the staff while they complete their tasks.

The impact of the treatment of people with advanced dementia

People with dementia are as affected as anyone by how they are regarded and treated by others. Learned helplessness theory (Seligman, 1972) refers to the emotional state experienced when one perceives a lack of control over one's situation or environment. Consequently, individuals resign themselves to this negative view and accept their supposed ineffectiveness. Lubinski (1995) applied learned helplessness theory to dementia to illuminate both the experience of dementia and attitudes towards it. For example, when people with dementia perceive that their communicative bids and responses are ineffectual, they stop engaging. The emotive and now generally discouraged term 'socially dead' (Sweeting and Gilhooly, 1997) was introduced to describe the way people with dementia who cannot speak are viewed. This occurs when people in the surrounding environment regard the person with dementia, although still physically alive, as socially inept, unworthy and effectively dead in respect of participation in the social world.

The perception of individuals with dementia as 'inept', 'dead', 'unworthy' and so on reflects negative attitudes towards them, how we feel about them and, ultimately, how we treat them. As Kitwood (1997) suggested, we 'dehumanise' people with dementia with our approach and opinions, and this is not only related to our cultural inheritance. Perhaps even more shockingly, we dehumanise individuals with dementia to protect *ourselves* from the reality of advanced dementia. At first glance, this behaviour seems callous, unfeeling and self-serving. However, caregivers *must* find ways of protecting themselves from 'burning out' as the job is extremely physically and emotionally draining. We need alternative ways of helping carers to cope with the psychological demands of their jobs that protect them and the people they care for. Perhaps, counterintuitively, this might involve getting *closer to* rather than distancing themselves from individuals with dementia. However, this development of relationships becomes extremely challenging when speech is no longer a viable means of communication. How, then, can we achieve an unspoken connection?

Kitwood (1997, p. 75) said, 'In the course of dementia a person will try to use whatever resources he or she still has available. If some of the more sophisticated means of action have dwindled away, it may be necessary to fall back on ways that are more basic, and more deeply learned; some of these were learned in early childhood.' As such, some people with dementia exhibit persistent bodily movements, which often involve the stimulation of their own bodies, such as rubbing their leg, chewing their fingers, pulling at items of their clothing or patting either themselves or external objects with their hands (Kitwood, 1997). Perrin (2001) proposed that these behaviours should be regarded as self-stimulatory in nature and occur in response to the failure of the environment to provide the person with dementia with occupation and a feeling of security.

As such, the person with dementia retreats into their own world and these repetitive behaviours provide stimulation that possibly represents a 'last desperate bid to remain psychologically alive' (Kitwood, 1997, p. 75). These self-stimulatory behaviours may potentially be used as a basis of communication between people with severe dementia and their caregivers.

Improving communication

There are multiple examples of interventions that have been developed to improve communication between individuals living with early to mid-stage dementia and their family members and professional caregivers, such as the Communication Enhancement Model (Orange et al., 1995) and FOCUSED (Ripich, 1994). However, there are far fewer suggested interventions when it comes to improving communication between people with more advanced dementia and those who care for them. Here we consider two: validation therapy (Feil, 1993) and habilitation therapy (Raia, 2011), both of which speak to the personhood of the individual.

Validation therapy

Validation therapy (Feil, 1993) was developed in the late 1960s as a means of communicating with older people and was directed towards individuals with dementia in the 1980s (Neal and Barton-Wright, 2003). Validation therapy is based on recognising and validating the individual's subjective reality. As such, even if the caregiver cannot understand the communication of the individual with dementia, they must act as though they do. In so doing, the caregiver does not attempt to orientate the person with dementia to present reality; rather they attempt to enter the world of the person with dementia. This principle serves to validate the subjective experience of the person with dementia, thereby valuing that person's emotions. Feil (1993) outlined a set of validation principles for caregivers to follow that embody the main thrust of validation therapy. For example, all behaviour engaged in by people with dementia must be regarded as having a meaning behind it and the person cannot be forced to change their behaviour. Caregivers are also encouraged to accept each individual non-judgementally and to view all people with dementia as valuable, no matter how much cognitive deterioration they have experienced.

Feil (1993) noted several ostensible benefits of validation for people with dementia, including improvements in speech, facial expression, communication with others and reduced need for the use of physical restraints or drugs. However, there is a lack of scientific evidence in support of its effectiveness, particularly regarding how changes are measured (Neal and Barton-Wright, 2003). Despite this, the basic principles of validation therapy – maintaining and validating the individual – in themselves suggest that the techniques employed might evoke positive emotion and enhance self-esteem. These in turn would also have a positive impact on quality of life. Moreover, validation therapy views the whole person, someone with a personal and emotional history, and attempts to maximise the retained abilities of individuals, in accordance with person-centredness.

Habilitation therapy

Habilitation therapy (Raia, 2011) represents a way of thinking that is geared towards improving the quality of life for people with advanced dementia by enhancing their confidence and functional abilities. The name is a deliberate attempt to make a distinction between therapies that focus on *re*habilitating the cognitive changes of dementia and this approach, which attempts to work with people with dementia as they are. 'The goal of habilitation therapy is deceptively simple: to bring about a positive emotion and to maintain that emotional state over the course of the day' (Raia, 2011, p. 2). It rests on caregiver perceptions of the person with dementia and their maintained psychological function; namely their ability to experience and communicate emotions, and aims to better understand the global impact of dementia as a whole. As such, habilitation therapy attempts to gain insight into how individuals with advanced dementia communicate and experience the communicative bids of others (Raia, 1999). Raia and Koenig-Coste (1996) described five domains where there are opportunities for positive emotion. These are: the physical domain, social domain, communication domain, functional domain and behavioural domain.

The physical domain focuses on identifying and addressing factors in the environment that can cause distress or confusion to people with dementia. This can include restructuring activities within the environment or making physical changes such as enhanced lighting (Raia, 2011).

Within the social domain, the goal is to facilitate the person with dementia to maintain social and cognitive skills via caregiver practice. As such, the caregiver is encouraged to work with and to maximise the retained verbal and nonverbal communication skills of the person with dementia. The main desired outcome of this approach is to encourage expression of positive emotions through having a sense of purpose and engagement in a meaningful activity. Within the realm of communication, habilitation therapy aims to facilitate mutual understanding between people with dementia and their caregivers. The desired outcome is to reduce frustration due to the verbal difficulties of the person with dementia, thereby encouraging the use of all retained communication skills for longer. The use of habilitation therapy in the communication domain requires the caregiver to listen intently and to be extremely creative and encouraging. In so doing, the caregiver must endeavour not so much to make sense of the verbal output of the person with dementia but, rather, the emotional message behind it. Furthermore, the caregiver must use and encourage the use of nonverbal communication as a method of facilitating retained communicative abilities in the person with dementia. In the functional domain, the goal is to prevent excess disability, a major problem for people with dementia who become disabled by the environment. The behavioural domain promotes a person-centred approach to care, assisting caregivers to identify things they can change in themselves or the environment.

Nonverbal communication

CHRISSIE

Chrissie spends a lot of time alone in Roseford Care Home, often in her room. She can no longer walk or independently get out of bed and is reliant on other people coming to see her or for staff to get her up and into a wheelchair so she can go out into the unit with other people. However, this does not happen very often as she frequently makes a loud, high-pitched sound apparently for no reason. This can be unsettling to the people around her as it sounds like she is in pain or distress and as such she is often left out of social activities. Her daughter, Jean, visits most days and always finds her mum to be very tactile and responsive. She is upset that Chrissie spends so much time alone in her room and encourages the staff to try to distract her by moving her bed or putting music on. When they run out of ideas and Jean goes home, the door is often closed on Chrissie and she eventually falls asleep. The carers are at a loss as to how to interact with Chrissie and they would love to find a way of connecting with her.

When people with dementia are no longer able to speak, this poses a significant problem, not only in terms of the obvious barriers to communication that this contributes to but also how it affects the way in which we 'see' those living with the condition.

For example, Duffy (1999) argued that caregivers of people with dementia have an 'intuitive dependence on language as a sign of emotional connection' (p. 577). In other words, when a person loses the ability to produce and to understand speech, we are likely to feel emotionally distant from them. Furthermore, we may feel that the person is incapable of connecting with us if they cannot express their feelings via speech. This may sound harsh but it is a situation that many people with dementia who cannot speak find themselves in. They are often ignored or avoided because we instinctively feel as though there is 'no-one there'. On a more positive note, Duffy (1999) also asserted that our internal experience of the world is not made up of language alone and that there are other ways of understanding human communication. So, what might these be? Let's use a couple of different examples to start us thinking about other forms of communication and the ways in which we can connect with others on an emotional level without the need to use words.

PAUSE FOR THOUGHT: NONVERBAL COMMUNICATION

Imagine you are at the cinema with a friend, watching a sad movie – let's say, *Titanic*. The movie is nearly finished and Jack and Rose are having their final scene together. After an extremely emotional heart-to-heart, they finally let go of each other's hands and Jack drops slowly down into the freezing water, never to be seen again. Now, imagine you hear a 'sniff' coming from the direction of your friend – what do you assume that indicates? You are in the dark and you can't see her but you know she's crying. You know this because not only did she make a sound associated with crying, you are tuned in to the emotion she is feeling. You are immediately able to connect with that feeling – not because she has told you she is upset but because her behaviour has 'told' you. This has happened in perhaps a more visceral way: you 'feel' it more than if she had said, 'I am upset.' Almost without thinking, you reach out for her hand and give it a squeeze. What does this 'say' to your friend? It says something that may be extremely difficult to put into words, but the 'feeling' is clear – perhaps even more so than if you'd spoken to her.

This idea of behaviour as communication is not a new one. As we saw in our *Titanic* example, nonverbal methods can often communicate the subtext of an interaction. As social beings, we are innately attuned to these cues and, as such, we attend subconsciously to nonverbal signals such as kinesics (bodily movement), tacesics (touch) and proxemics (orientation and spacing) (Bull, 2002). Kinesics refers to several aspects of nonverbal behaviour relating to movements including posture, body movements, gestures, eye gaze and facial expressions (Shea, 1998). Proxemics on the other hand is specifically concerned with how the distance between two people affects their behaviour and relationship (Shea, 1998). In his analysis, Shea (1998) also referred to 'paralanguage' as the aspects of communication that include prosody, rate, rhythm, volume, tone and pitch of voice.

It has been estimated that 60–65 per cent of our communication is nonverbal (Burgoon, Guerrero and Floyd, 2009). Albert Mehrabian in his 1971 book *Silent Messages* highlighted the central importance of nonverbal communication in human interactions and the multiple messages we convey. For instance, if we feel uncomfortable and want to end a conversation we turn away from the person we are speaking to and break eye contact (Mehrabian, 1971). Other research has demonstrated the ways that nonverbal behaviours work in combination. For example, Burgoon et al. (1984) manipulated eye gaze, proximity, body lean, smiling and touch in an experiment with 150 participants. They found that 'high eye contact, close proximity, forward body lean, and smiling, all conveyed greater intimacy, attraction and trust. Low eye contact, a distal position, backward body lean, and the absence of smiling and touch communicated greater detachment' (Burgoon et al., 1984, p. 351).

Now let's look at another example of nonverbal communication and our amazing ability to interpret, translate and to 'feel' it. Imagine this time that you are visiting a friend who has a two-month-old baby. After a short while, your friend asks you if you wouldn't mind looking after the baby for 20 minutes while he pops out to the shop. You have never had a baby of your own and are more than a little apprehensive about what 'to do' with her. However, you agree to look after her while your friend runs an errand.

The moment your friend leaves the house, you start to feel self-conscious and doubtful as to your ability to care for the infant. However, she is asleep and you sit down to wait for your friend to return. Then you hear a sound from the crib and realise the baby is waking up. She makes a sound and you get a little closer to see what she is doing. The baby immediately spots you and you smile at her – quite instinctively. She responds to you with a smile. You smile again and she keeps looking at you and smiling. Then you repeat the sound she made and she keeps her eyes on yours. Then you try another sound and she keeps looking and she makes a sound. Then you smile again and the two of you are having a 'conversation'. However, you don't feel that you need to speak to the baby. Nevertheless, what you both understand from this exchange is that you are interested in each other, are happy to be together and have, in some way, connected. Just like the cinema example, the communication that you have engaged in with the baby is more about 'feeling' something than conveying a message. You have communicated without words on perhaps a deeper level than you might if you could talk to each other.

Now imagine a situation where you find yourself alone in a room with a person with dementia in an advanced stage. The lady is lying in bed with her eyes open, appearing to stare into space. She is gently pulling at the top of her blanket, over and over in a rhythmic motion, and is making a loud humming noise. How do you think you would feel in this situation? Would you feel curious like you did with your friend's baby and approach the lady? Would you try to gain her attention? To make eye contact? To touch the hand that is pulling the blanket? Would you start humming too? Our experience tells us probably not.

What would you make of her actions? Would you feel awkward, unsure, concerned? Probably. What if you were to approach the lady and try to interact with her in some way? How would you even begin? What might you expect to happen? How might she respond? Would she hit out? Would she shout? Would she ignore you? Would you be embarrassed? Would you feel as though you had failed? Now, would you have asked yourself *any* of those questions in response to the cinema and baby examples? Again, probably not. Why do we feel this way about interacting with people with dementia who cannot use words? There are many different reasons why we might be apprehensive or embarrassed about trying to interact with someone with dementia. However, if we are to attempt to help these individuals to reconnect to the social world, we need to put our own concerns aside and focus on what the person needs.

STACEY
Stacey is the manager of Roseford Care Home and she finds caring for Chrissie perplexing. Chrissie appears to be happy when she is with people. However, the high-pitched sound she makes causes concern to other residents and their visitors, but also to many of the staff. Because Chrissie is unable to walk she is totally reliant on staff getting her up and out of bed. Stacey finds that some of them are more

comfortable than others to take her out of her room due to the sound she makes. When Chrissie's daughter Jean comes to visit, she is sad and disappointed to find her mum alone in her room and asks Stacey if she can ensure that if her mum is not participating in group activities, someone at least spends time every day interacting with her one-to-one. Stacey would like Chrissie to participate in the social activities on the unit but cannot see a way to achieve this without upsetting other residents or their families.

It may be the case that you have worked with individuals like Chrissie, Eleanor and Bert for many years and feel that you know what 'they' are like. You might think that there is no point in trying to engage with someone in this situation as they seem unaware of what is going on around them. You may have no idea as to how you might even begin to connect with a person with dementia who cannot speak. Throughout this book, you will learn about why people feel the way they do towards individuals with advanced dementia. More importantly, you will learn how to reframe these feelings in a way that will afford both you and the person/people you care for to engage in meaningful interaction. This is Adaptive Interaction.

Summary

The impact of dementia on communication is complex and is influenced by the specific effects of neurodegeneration interacting with environmental, especially social, factors. Clearly, as dementia progresses, although people experience many identifiable difficulties there is equally a range of retained functions. If it were possible to develop these remaining skills, the probability of mutually rewarding interactions occurring between people with dementia and their caregivers could be improved. Consequently, any intervention that aims to promote communication in people with dementia must target these relatively intact functions (Azuma and Bayles, 1997). As we have seen, focusing on speech-based activities can be helpful for improving communication with people with mild to moderate dementia. However, for people with dementia who have little or no retained speech, nonverbal strategies must be used to achieve mutually meaningful interactions. These possibilities are explored in the following chapters.

Chapter 3

I Hear You Now

Collaborative Communication

This chapter introduces the collaborative communication model to help you to understand the roles of the communication partners in two-way interactions. You will learn about the fundamentals of communication and their role in language development. The notion of individuals with additional communication support needs is also introduced, including pre-speech infants, people with severe autism and people with advanced dementia, all illustrated with examples.

Human communication

As mentioned in Chapter 1, humans are characteristically social beings and as such, strive to communicate as soon as they enter the world (Meltzoff and Moore, 1983; Valenza et al., 1996). Through communication with others we share information about ourselves and each other which is ultimately essential to our survival (MacDonald and Leary, 2005). For example, a newborn infant cries when hungry and his parents quickly learn to respond to this cue by providing him with food. Without this type of basic communication, the infant's chances of survival would be greatly reduced.

Infant communication

Although communicative bids in infants are undoubtedly primitive, they are nevertheless evident from the moment of birth, often in the form of imitative behaviours. Babies are born equipped to respond to human faces (Valenza et al., 1996) and can mimic simple facial activities, such as sticking out the tongue (Meltzoff and Moore, 1983). Such imitative behaviours suggest that humans have an innate predisposition to communicate and interact with others. Parents of newborns typically repeat and reinforce the facial expressions, sounds and movements made by their infants without being aware of it. This imitation forms the basis of their early interactions and provides the foundation for future communication. In parent–infant interactions this reciprocal behaviour arises quite naturally and is both spontaneous and unselfconscious (Tomasello, 1992).

BERT'S PERSPECTIVE
Bert awakes and opens his eyes. He looks around but does not know where he is. He wants to get out of bed and walk Isla but he cannot seem to move. He tries to call out but nothing seems to happen. He can hear sounds but does not recognise them. After a while Bert feels tired and closes his eyes again. He misses Isla and being out in the woods but he feels tired all the time.

Infants' communication skills develop by engaging with their parents in this early 'protoconversation' and continue to improve with their support and encouragement (Papoušek, 1995). Indeed, it is commonly thought that *all* cognitive skills, including language and self-awareness, stem from social interactions with more skilled individuals (Haden, 1998). Known as 'scaffolding', parents facilitate the development of language and self-awareness by interacting with their babies as if their early communicative bids make sense to them (Newson, 1978). You will undoubtedly have engaged in this sort of 'as if' interaction with an infant at some point, probably without realising its significance. For example, when a baby 'babbles' you might respond by saying, 'Oh, are you telling me a story?' The baby babbles again and you say, 'Really? And *then* what happened?' This type of interaction allows infants to communicate with their parents in a way that although primitive, is nevertheless full of meaning to them both (Vygotsky, 1978). Consequently, infants become increasingly aware of their effect on others and of their status as increasingly skilled communicators.

Human communication fulfils numerous vitally important functions essential to human survival. In evolutionary terms, social animals that were well integrated into their family groups and formed strong bonds with other animals were more likely to survive than those that did not seek out the company of others. In other words, 'for social animals, being socially excluded was often equivalent to death' (MacDonald and Leary, 2005, p. 203). Although perhaps less imminently life-threatening in today's world, the effect of social exclusion has a major negative impact on a person's existence. Indeed, the impact of social rejection is regarded to be *so* significant that it has even been related to physical pain and is thought to be controlled by the same physiological system (MacDonald and Leary, 2005).

PAUSE FOR THOUGHT: THE PITFALLS OF SOCIAL MEDIA

As of July 2017, there are over 1.94 billion monthly active Facebook users worldwide (Zephoria Digital Marketing, 2017). The popularity of Facebook is undeniable and it has become part of our daily vocabulary and lives. Facebook's main benefit is that it can both keep us connected to those we already know and help us to make new connections. The platform can make it easy to check in with family who live on the other side of the world, reconnect with old school friends or, in some cases, meet new partners. However, there is also a dark side to Facebook. It is a haven for cyber bullying and adults as well as teenagers and children have been known to fall prey to this cruel phenomenon. Not quite so serious but emotionally salient nonetheless, Facebook can sometimes make us feel excluded. Here's an example:

You login to Facebook on Monday morning to find an album of photos from a birthday party that took place over the weekend. The photos show a group of your friends having fun, celebrating a birthday – but *you* were not invited. You read your friends' comments, saying what a great night they had and how happy they were to have been there.

How do you feel? Do you experience a lurch in the pit of your stomach when you see the post? You might possibly have lots of questions you would like to ask your friends as to why you were not invited. A range of reasons as to why you were not included may be running through your mind. 'Did I annoy someone?', 'Does someone dislike me?', 'Have they gone off me?'

Whatever you are *telling* yourself at that moment, you are most likely *feeling* rejected. Now, you are experiencing something like what social exclusion might feel like for a person living with dementia who cannot speak. The world goes on around you, yet you are playing no part in it. It hurts and there is nothing you can do about it.

Personhood and intersubjectivity

Personhood is the experience of being a person, which is co-created through co-operation with one or more other individuals. Essentially other people treat you as a fellow human being by interacting with you. Infants are attributed personhood through interaction with parents (Vygotsky, 1978). The attribution of 'personhood' to an individual represents an affirmation of their status as a person in every sense of the word. However, personhood is socially constructed, co-created and maintained by relationships that encourage effective and supportive communication (Kitwood and Bredin, 1992).

BETTY'S PERSPECTIVE

Betty and Frank have always tried speaking when they are with Bert even though he does not respond. They try to include him in the conversation but he shows no reaction, he does not make any sounds or eye contact and they wonder if he can hear them. They had also thought he would respond to Isla but he is not able to move any more, to reach down and pat her. They find it hard to keep visiting him but they still hold onto the memory of Bert their neighbour and hope that they can make a connection with him or that he at least knows they are there.

Personhood is intrinsically linked to the concept of 'intersubjectivity' which refers to our innate human ability to comprehend and appreciate each other (Rommetveit, 1974). Rommetveit (1974) argued that even the simplest communicative act rests upon the participants' 'mutual commitment to a shared social world' (p. 29). In other words, intersubjectivity is something we achieve together without explicit discussion. Trevarthen (2004) proposed that for this to be possible, we must regard all human action as communicative.

From this point of view we can more easily understand how communication developed and how infants and parents first begin to interact. To discuss communication as both a collaborative act and one that is vital to human life requires a framework that encompasses these concepts and considers them as interdependent. There are many models of interpersonal communication and a full review is out of scope of this book. However, we briefly consider the difference between monologic and dialogic models of interpersonal communication to highlight the relative roles of each interaction partner.

Models of communication

Monologic models of interpersonal communication

Monologic models of communication refer to the types of interactions where communicators are far more interested in themselves than in the relationship between them (Buber, 1958). In monologic communication one person speaks while the other listens and there is no real interaction between them. The communication is one-directional and the speaker has little or no interest in the other person. He or she may be reluctant to listen to the other person as the purpose is for the speaker to convey their message, not to engage in a dialogue. The speaker may even be critical or make negative comments towards the other person.

However, human social exchange is a 'joint accomplishment' by partners who have a shared communicative goal in mind. As such, the meanings of the messages in the conversation are dependent upon the social situation within which they are exchanged. Subsequently, the separate inputs of the communicator and listener do not hold the same meaning (Krauss, 2005). This type of communication can be seen in care settings where a caregiver is giving instructions or information but not expecting a reply from the person they are speaking to.

Dialogic models of communication

As in the monologic models, the dialogic approach views speech as the main method of communication, but it differs significantly in how it regards the goal of the communication. According to the dialogic models, the goal of the interaction is not simply to exchange information, as in the monologic models, but to achieve 'intersubjectivity' or mutual understanding. In dialogic models of interaction, each person plays the role of listener and speaker, and both communication partners show a genuine regard for and seek to understand the experiences of the other. There is a deep concern and respect for the other person and the relationship between them in this type of communication. Dialogic communicators avoid negative criticism and negative personal judgement and they show a willingness to listen to each other. The listeners and speakers can make their own choices and use nonverbal cues to indicate their involvement.

The collaborative model

One example of a dialogic model is Clark and Brennan's (1991) collaborative theory. Clark and Brennan proposed that communication amounts to much more than the exchange of spoken messages between conversational partners. Rather, they regarded communication as a collaborative effort in that both partners seek to work with and understand each other (Figure 3.1.). For example, should a misunderstanding arise in a conversation, both partners will attempt to resolve it.

By engaging in this process, both partners work to expend the 'least collaborative effort' (Clark and Wilkes-Gibbs, 1986). In other words, one partner might make an extra effort to minimise the collective effort made by both Clark and Brennan (1991). This form of joint endeavour represents the basis for facilitative interaction with individuals who have additional communication needs. However, for this process to begin the communicator without additional needs must first regard all the other individual's actions as intentionally communicative.

We have previously illustrated collaborative communication in terms of parent–infant interaction. This is a relatively easy example to understand as it is likely to be one that we have had experience of either engaging in or witnessing. However, let's now consider an example that we may not have encountered before – one that perhaps might seem a little unusual – where we also become individuals with additional communication needs.

Imagine you are a secondary school pupil who attends a mainstream comprehensive school. The school also contains a class of around a dozen pupils who are profoundly deaf. Hearing and hearing-impaired pupils are integrated during physical education classes but they don't mix well as they don't understand each other's languages. Your teacher comes up with a plan that every Monday, hearing-impaired and hearing pupils are to be paired up and do their lessons together with two teachers – one who signs and one who speaks. Your teacher believes that this is a good idea so that you and your classmates can get to know and understand each other. You are paired with Isabella, a profoundly deaf teenager who doesn't use speech to communicate but is expert in sign language. You wonder how on earth you will be able to interact with Isabella as you don't know any sign language. Your teachers give you a task to complete together – you must design a car that you can both drive with features that are useful to each of you. This seems like a difficult task for you and Isabella to achieve – how will you ever be able to 'talk' to each other? The answer is that you have to try to collaborate, to find some middle ground – to find a language that you will both understand. In the case of you and Isabella, it's relatively easy to see that you are able to write to each other. You scribble ideas on paper and pass them between you. You even use your 'own' sign language at times by displaying facial expressions and bodily movements to indicate agreement (thumbs-up), disagreement (shaking the head), uncertainty (shrugging the shoulders). You pass a pen between you and take turns in writing down your ideas and questions for each other. You are working together to expend the least effort.

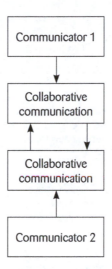

Figure 3.1 Representation of Clark and Brennan's (1991) collaborative model

Individuals with additional communication needs

Earlier in this chapter we outlined how healthy infants enter the social world. It is possible to view infants as individuals with additional communication needs in that they attempt to communicate in an environment that is dominated by speech – a form of communication they have yet to comprehend and use. However, as facilitative 'protoconversation' increases between infants and their parents, they slowly begin to develop an understanding of and an ability to use language. Thus healthy infants have additional communication needs for a relatively short period of their lives and are quickly accepted as social agents (see Figure 3.2).

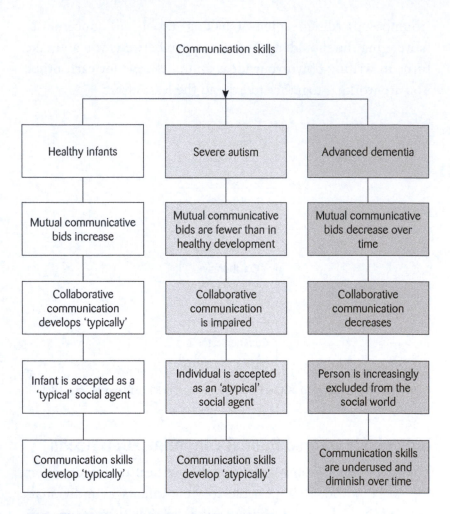

Figure 3.2 The trajectory of communication skills in communicators with additional needs

Individuals with severe autism very often experience profound communication difficulties from birth. As such, the communication skills of infants and children with autism spectrum disorders (ASD) tend to develop 'atypically' and often these individuals never become able to use recognisable speech at all. Getting to grips with the social world is not an easy task for individuals living with ASD, as the supportive communication that develops between healthy infants and children and their parents is typically impaired owing both to cognitive difficulties experienced by the person with ASD and the inability of his parents to communicate in a way that is meaningful to him. Consequently, the individual with severe ASD is regarded as an 'atypical' social agent (see Figure 3.2). Indeed, for a long time it was believed that individuals with severe ASD lacked the drive to communicate with others altogether (Hobson, 1993). However, work by Nadel and others has demonstrated that not only can people with ASD participate in social situations; they also have awareness of others as separate individuals and a demonstrable urge to interact and communicate. This latter point was illuminated through the 'still face' paradigm, a controversial manipulation of the social situation that involves the interaction partner ceasing the interaction part way through to see what the other person does (Nadel, 2000).

ELEANOR'S PERSPECTIVE

Eleanor is nearly always in pain. People seem to come out of nowhere and move her around. She doesn't see them at first, then suddenly there they are standing over her. Why are there so many of them? She wants to tell the people to leave her alone when they take a hold of her like that. They lift her up and her arms and legs fall and twist and it hurts. Everything hurts – all over and she's terrified of being touched. She can't tell them to stay away so she tries to warn anyone who comes near her by other means. She stares at them and moves her mouth to try to speak but nothing comes out. When that doesn't work, she tries to fend them off with her arms and legs.

People whose communication skills are compromised as the result of dementia have a different experience from infants and children with ASD, although all can be regarded as communicators with additional needs. The main difference is that infants and children with ASD are trying to enter the social world while people with dementia are attempting to maintain their grip on it. For these groups of communicators with additional needs, the role of the communication partner is crucial to their development or performance. In other words, communication will fail if the partner with a full set of communication skills does not facilitate the interaction by working to expend the 'least collaborative effort' (Clark and Wilkes-Gibb, 1986). It becomes the task of the interaction partner to 'use (his) creativity to establish a new channel of communication' (Kitwood, 1997, p. 3).

Communication by individuals with dementia is also different from infants and children with ASD as their skills and needs are constantly changing as dementia progresses (Figure 3.2). Also, unlike these other groups, most people with dementia were previously able to communicate expertly and functioned in the human social world without any major difficulties.

JAMES' PERSPECTIVE

James finds it challenging to even think about communicating with Eleanor. She is thought to be 'difficult' to deal with and he has heard stories from his colleagues about being hit by her. She often throws people 'dirty looks' and screws up her face when people talk to her. How is he supposed to interact with someone who clearly doesn't want to? He tries to imagine how she might be feeling and wonders if she can understand how he feels too. He thinks she doesn't want to communicate, but why? On the other hand, Eleanor thinks James is there to cause her pain, but why? How can they ever know what the other is feeling?

Improving interpersonal communication between people with dementia and their caregivers could improve both the job satisfaction of care staff and the quality of life of people with dementia (Woods, 1999). A combination of the retained communicative behaviours of the person with dementia and facilitative interaction by the caregiver could form the basis of interventions designed specifically for dementia. In short, collaborative communication represents the crucial area that may well have the potential to enhance the lives of people with dementia and those who care for them.

Intensive Interaction

Although speech-based interactions eventually become unfeasible for people with very severe dementia, this does not mean that they have lost the urge or capacity to communicate (Astell and Ellis, 2006; Ellis and Astell, 2004, 2008). Intensive Interaction is an intervention that was developed in the 1980s to facilitate communication between people with severe and profound learning disabilities and their caregivers. The focus of II is on regular nonverbal and subvocal exchanges with little or no involvement of speech. In II the quality of the interaction is all-important and there is no emphasis on contents, task performance or achieving specific outcomes (Nind, 1996). The key to II is that the behaviour of the nonverbal participant is viewed as intentionally communicative.

The principles of II are based on the fundamental building blocks that develop communication between infants and their parents. For example, as soon as they are born, babies strive to communicate with other people by, for example, imitating facial expressions and bodily movements (Meltzoff and Moore, 1983). Babies and their parents later imitate each other's facial expression, movements and sounds quite naturally and it is this type of interaction that precedes the development of language. As such, mutual imitation of behaviour is a key element of II. Although the structure and the linguistic contents of these early exchanges are nonverbal, it is difficult to argue that they are without meaning or emotion (Papoušek, 1995). Furthermore, the extrapolation of principles from the earliest communication exchanges does not mean that people with learning disabilities or, by extension, other severe communication impairments should be regarded or treated as if they were infants (Nind, 1999).

When engaging in II with a person with severe and profound learning disabilities, it is essential to identify and work with each person's individual communicative repertoire (Caldwell, 2005). Nind (1999) suggests that the communication partner take some time to become familiar with the person they will be working with to assess which types of behaviours they might engage in. This initial 'connection' is then developed by the communication partner into a set of spontaneous interactive 'games' that are based on the behaviour of the person with communication impairment. For example, a sound or action they make, such as banging on the table, might be reflected by their partner, either directly or with some variation in the rhythm. The professional or caregiver responds contingently to their partner's behaviours to continuously expand the interaction between them and support their partner to take a more active role in communication.

Some practitioners consider the focus of II to be on teaching the 'pre-speech fundamentals' of communication such as turn-taking, shared attention, and eye gaze (e.g. Hewett, 1996; Nind, 1999). These practitioners term the professional or caregiver the 'teacher' and the communication-impaired partner the 'learner'. Through constant modification of their own interpersonal behaviours, to make them as engaging and as meaningful as possible to their partner with additional communication needs, the teacher attempts to build up the fundamental elements of communication.

In a contrasting approach to II, Caldwell (2005) views the caregiver or professional as the learner, attempting to 'learn the language' of their partner. In Caldwell's approach imitation is the starting point of II: 'a way of capturing attention, a door to enter the inner world of our partners' (Caldwell, 2008, p. 176). One key outcome of this approach is providing a way for people typically regarded as outside the social world to express themselves (Caldwell and Horwood, 2007). By responding in ways that are familiar to the person with severe communication difficulties, that is, initially imitating and then developing them into a shared 'language', it is possible to build and sustain close relationships with people who cannot speak (Caldwell, 2005).

CHRISSIE'S PERSPECTIVE

Chrissie is more than capable of communicating, although most others do not see it that way. She wants to cuddle and laugh and sing but no-one stops to sit with her. There is a lot of noise in the background that is getting louder and louder. Chrissie starts singing over the top of it and she soon finds herself on her own again. When she is in the dining room and tries to start a sing-song, she is whisked away once more. When she is feeling bored in the dayroom and sings to herself for her own amusement, she is taken back to her room and put to bed. Singing is all she has left and no-one wants to join in with her.

Studies using II typically employ video recording to measure developments in communicative responses (e.g. Kellett, 2000, 2003; Nind, 1996). For example, Nind (1996) examined a range of basic communication behaviours, including smiling, eye contact and looking at the communication partner's face. Caldwell uses video recording both to learn her partner's 'language' and also to teach caregivers how to use this language in their interactions (Caldwell, 2005). II has been shown to increase communication behaviours (Samuel and Maggs, 1998) and improve quality of life in people with severe and profound learning disabilities (Rayner et al., 2014). Improved quality of life is commonly seen in shifts from solitary self-stimulatory behaviour, such as biting or head banging, to engagement in shared activity (Caldwell and Horwood, 2007; Coia and Jardine Handley, 2008). The actual contents of the interaction are not important, as the aim of II is not to convey or to exchange information. Rather, the main objective of II is to allow people with severe and profound learning disabilities to simply connect with another human being. We felt strongly that the principles of this approach held promise for people with very severe dementia who are typically excluded from social interactions.

Using Intensive Interaction with people with dementia

Our first attempt at using the principles of II was with Jessie, a lady who had been living with dementia for a number of years, but who still retained some speech. Jessie constantly walked around the care home talking to herself and to anyone who would listen and she often appeared to be upset. Based on their experience, staff members advised us that Jessie was unlikely to sit down and engage in an interaction. To get to know Jessie, Maggie (first author) joined her in walking around the care home. Contrary to the concerns expressed by the staff, Jessie showed a great willingness to sit and interact with Maggie for periods up to half an hour. She demonstrated a retained desire to interact by communicating with Maggie through speech, extended eye contact and facial expressions that indicated interest (Ellis and Astell, 2004). In keeping with Kitwood's (1997) proposal, she used the most sophisticated means of communication that were available to her. Specifically, although Jessie's speech was muddled and difficult for her communication partner to understand, she favoured it as her main mode of interaction. However, it was the *combination* of words, sounds, facial expressions and eye contact that constituted her personal language. To interact with Jessie, it was necessary for Maggie to learn and to use this language to the best of her ability. She then reflected Jessie's words and communicative behaviours back in a way that was meaningful to Jessie.

Encouraged by this preliminary work we completed a case study using the principles of II in a more systematic way with Edie, a lady with dementia who could no longer speak. We were interested in identifying Edie's completely nonverbal communicative repertoire. This involved spending time in the care home to piece together a picture of (i) the communication that took place between caregivers and Edie, (ii) the opportunities for communication that occurred during any given day, and (iii) Edie's repertoire of communication skills. The observational part of the study reflected the findings of Bowie and Mountain's (1993) observation conducted on an in-patient unit for people with dementia where they found people spent up to two-thirds of their time engaged in no activity at all, social or otherwise. In Edie's case, she spent most of her time alone in her room, with caregivers going in for short periods only to carry out specific care tasks. The communication that took place was brief, perfunctory and consisted largely of questions such as, 'Have you seen the weather today?' or 'Did you eat your breakfast?' to which Edie was unable to respond with speech.

We used these findings to construct what we termed a baseline or 'Standard Interaction', comprising a set of questions based on those listed above. Maggie spent ten minutes with Edie, working through the questions and allowing 20 seconds after each for Edie to respond nonverbally. Maggie then spent another ten minutes with Edie, using the principles of II to learn Edie's language and engage in a dialogue with her. Using the principles of II, we found that Edie had a rich communication repertoire, comprising sound, movement, directed eye gaze, touch and facial expressions (Ellis and Astell, 2008). Edie was extremely eager to interact with Maggie and appeared to revel in the opportunity to make meaningful human contact. This was evident by the fact that Edie laughed at several points. She also reached out to touch and rub heads with Maggie during the II session while not using any of these behaviours during the Standard Interaction session.

Based on these two case studies, we felt that this approach had potential to improve the lives of people with dementia who can no longer speak, their family members and professional caregivers by providing them with a platform for communication not reliant on speech. However, we recognised that we would be going against deep-rooted misconceptions about people with dementia who cannot speak: that they cannot, and have no desire to, communicate (Duffy, 1999; Kitwood, 1997). Therefore, we also wanted to explore further the communication environment as it became clear from our work both with Jessie and Edie that the perceptions and attitudes of caregivers, who were their main communication partners, were a crucial component of the interaction. If caregivers believed that an individual had few or no retained communication skills, this severely hampered their opportunities for interaction. Therefore, we were eager to explore the potential of II as a tool for communicating with all people living with dementia who can no longer speak. This would enable caregivers to communicate with and establish meaningful relationships with everyone they care for, irrespective of whether they can speak or not.

Adaptive Interaction

As stated above, Adaptive Interaction (AI) grew out of our training and understanding of II. The focus on making a connection with a person with additional communication needs resonated with our analysis of the communication experience of people with dementia who cannot speak. By making nonverbal communication central and focusing on the quality of the interaction, they could be afforded new opportunities for communication and participation in the social world.

STACEY'S PERSPECTIVE

Stacey wants to find a way to connect with Chrissie and involve her in social activities. She can see that Chrissie is eager to interact and seems to love being around other people. If Chrissie could only talk instead of making that noise, people would want to interact with her more often. Stacey has the perspective of someone with a full range of communicative abilities at her fingertips. As such, she understands 'effective' or 'proper' communication between people as something that is based on the exchange of messages. For example, when she asks her son what he wants for dinner and he tells her he'd like a takeaway – *that's* communication. Stacey sees Chrissie's sound not as a form of communication but as a symptom of dementia.

Expansion of the interactions over time is one of the core elements of II with people who have intellectual disabilities or ASD. Building up a shared language transforms the life of the individual who cannot use words, by equipping them with a means of exercising control over their environment. Being able to participate equally in shared interactions also transforms other people's attitudes and the ways they behave towards the individual. Seeing an individual as a fellow participant in the social world and valuing their participation leads to deeper and more meaningful relationships.

We wanted to achieve this for people with dementia who can no longer use words. When we started using II principles with people who have dementia we found that we could not know if they remembered the previous interactions. We found that we needed to approach each encounter aiming to re-establish a connection but ready to adapt to however the individual communicated in that instance. Sometimes people who had a repertoire of sounds were silent. Others who had previously moved their hands might keep them under the bedcovers or a blanket on their lap. And yet others whose communication was dominated by eye gaze might close their eyes and not respond.

Having learnt their language, we could look for communicative behaviours to home in on and re-establish a connection. We could also try initiating connections using elements of their own repertoires, such as sounds or movements. Mainly we learnt to be open minded about each interaction. Although we had used the principles of II to communicate with Edie, we recognised that the memory problems typical in this population meant that she may not recall previous interactions when we saw her again. In other words, we were prepared for interactions to start anew each time. As such, the communication partner would be required to adapt to whichever communicative behaviours the person with dementia engaged in at any given point. We therefore named our approach 'Adaptive Interaction'.

In embarking on this approach we were very mindful of the need for respect and to preserve the dignity of the people with dementia who cannot speak. We were especially concerned about the explicit use of imitation as 'mockery', which can involve exaggerated imitation of a person's behaviour or speech, which is one of Kitwood's personal detractors. However, imitation in the form of mirroring is the basis for empathetic communication and is underpinned by mirror neurons. 'Neural mirroring solves the "problem of other minds" (how we can access and understand the minds of others) and makes intersubjectivity possible, thus facilitating social behavior' (Iacoboni, 2009, p. 653). Duffy (1999) argued that communicating with individuals with dementia who cannot speak 'allows us to nourish and continue their still existing rich emotional life' (p. 579).

Summary

Collaborative communication is a model of interaction that requires individuals to enter into each other's worlds. In order to understand each other, we must find a common ground, a shared reality, and the sheer determination to make a connection. As people with a full range of communication skills at our disposal, we are more than capable of interacting with individuals with additional communication needs. This requires us to both consider that communication is far more than just speech and that we might achieve a closer bond with someone without speech. The process of AI is a constant negotiation between two humans with an innate desire to communicate with each other.

Chapter 4

Let's Work Together

Learning the Language of Dementia

As introduced in Chapter 3, AI is an approach to communicating without words. The process involves several steps (Figure 4.1). First is a process of getting to know the person with dementia. Second is understanding the communication environment. Third is identifying an individual's unique communication repertoire. Fourth is using the individual's communication repertoire to make a connection with the person. Fifth is building on this connection to establish an ongoing relationship. Here we describe these steps before going on to work through them in the following three chapters with Chrissie, Eleanor and Bert.

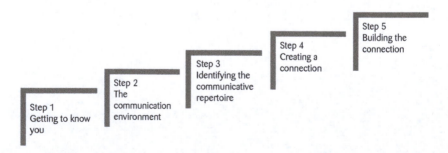

Figure 4.1 The Adaptive Interaction process

Templates of the assessment charts from this chapter are featured in the appendix, and are available to download and print from www.jkp.com/catalogue/book/9781785921971

Step 1: Getting to know you

The first step in the process is to assess how much information is already known about the person with dementia. This is best completed by the person or people who are going to be the communication partner or partners. The 'getting to know you' process involves gathering and combining information that is already known about the person with information which is found out through further investigation. This can be quite a fun process in terms of doing some detective work to find out about the person via their family and friends. However, it can also be upsetting in that it may highlight how little is known about the person. Moreover, if they do not have any regular visitors or family, it might not be possible to find out very much more than is already known. Nevertheless, this process is useful in helping to focus on the person, which is an important first step in being able to connect with them.

The Getting to Know You chart (Chart 4.1) captures both types of facts, i.e. those already known and those discovered through investigation. It also includes consideration of how the individual and the people they interact with are feeling. Recognising how we feel is important to address because social interaction and connection with other people are so important to being human. If one person is afraid or anxious or uncomfortable about interacting with another, then this can hamper any potential communication. It is also an important step in starting to consider the perspective of the person with dementia who cannot speak. What might it be like for them?

See below for an example of a chart completed by a formal caregiver about a person she cares for.

Getting to Know You	
How much personal information do you know about the person, e.g. previous occupation, number of children, hobbies?	Connie was a primary school teacher and loves children. She and her husband Paul couldn't have children, but they had several nieces and nephews they saw regularly. Connie enjoyed crafting, regularly going to evening classes to learn new skills.
What do you know about the person's life before he/she became ill?	Connie and Paul lived in a flat in the centre of town for over 40 years. Paul died a few years ago and Connie became unable to look after herself. She was diagnosed with dementia five years ago.
What are the person's likes and dislikes?	Connie's face lights up when she sees children. Her nephew Mat occasionally brings his little girl Izzie to see her and this always makes her smile.
What are the obstacles to communicating with this person?	I find it difficult to communicate with Connie as she can't speak and doesn't seem to understand what I'm saying to her either.
How do you think he/she might be currently feeling and why?	I think she feels lonely because she hardly ever has any visitors.
How do you feel when you try to interact with him/her and why?	I feel sad when I try to talk Connie as I feel I can't get through to her.

Chart 4.1 Sample Getting to Know You chart

Step 2: Communication environment

The communication environment refers to the physical and spatial aspects of where interactions take place (Knapp and Hall, 2010). For people living with dementia who can no longer speak we take a holistic and comprehensive view of the communication environment as encompassing the opportunities they have for communicating, the people who are available as communication partners, and the situations and contexts where communication takes place. Understanding when, where and with whom communication takes place is important for developing a strategy to implement and integrate AI into the daily lives of people living with dementia who cannot speak. The aims is for all potential communication partners to use nonverbal approaches in place of their default use of speech. Both at home or in a formal care settings this requires a concerted strategy from everyone to interact with individuals with dementia who can no longer speak in the most appropriate and meaningful way. Making these connections and being able to communicate will benefit all parties, enabling the development of closer and more rewarding caregiving relationships.

Opportunities for communication

As autonomous beings, we can choose to communicate as and when we please with whoever we please using whatever medium we choose. People with dementia who cannot speak have fewer opportunities to communicate as their ability to use a wide range of communication channels is reduced. At home and within care settings those who cannot walk rely on others to get them up, assist them into a wheelchair and take them out of their bedrooms. Opportunities for communication can occur during these activities. However, these may be largely *'functional'* in nature. What we mean by this is that the communication is focused on the task at hand– for example, helping someone to shower – and may not contain a social element.

Once outside their room people with dementia who can no longer speak may be taken to communal areas such as dining, sitting or activity areas. Here there may be a mixture of caregivers, visitors and other people with dementia. Again, these are all potential opportunities for communication and it is in these situations that there may be more opportunity for purely 'social' engagement. They may also be moving around the care setting, perhaps to the bathroom or, like Jessie, walking about. Others may spend time alone in their room reliant on other people to come to them.

An important element of implementing AI is that it be adopted as the communication channel for *every* interaction with individuals who can no longer speak. This means care partners recognising and taking all communication opportunities that occur and using AI rather than speech. AI should not be treated as a luxury, an add-on or special activity to be undertaken when caregivers have time to sit down and focus on an individual. It should be used in all encounters and situations with people who cannot speak, in a similar way to using sign language with people who are unable to hear.

Communication partners

As their social world shrinks people living with dementia who can no longer speak have limited numbers of people to communicate and interact with. For people who are still living at home, they are most likely to be interacting with family members. However, due to their additional needs, many people with dementia who can no longer speak live in long-term or nursing care settings. In this context, their most likely communication partners are staff who work in the care settings where they live. Alongside staff involved in direct care, this can include staff engaged in catering, cleaning, maintenance and administration. There may also be volunteers, families and other people with dementia. As such it is important to have a comprehensive understanding of all the people in the environment who can potentially interact with people with dementia who can no longer speak so they can all benefit from using nonverbal communication methods.

Communication situations and contexts

As we have already seen, many people living with dementia who can no longer speak also have accompanying challenges in daily life. This can include mobility problems which mean they cannot get out of bed independently, and walking may be difficult or no longer possible. They may also need assistance going to the toilet, bathing and eating. Our observations of the contexts and situations where communication mostly occurs identified that a large proportion of interactions take place during these activities of daily living. In our research, before we commence AI training, we ask caregivers to carry out a 'usual' interaction to provide a baseline for comparing AI against (see the section 'Observation of the communication environment' below). We find that most of these usual interactions involve an activity of daily living, particularly offering food or drink to the person with dementia who cannot speak. In many of these interactions, the staff spoke to the person with dementia, describing what they were doing such as 'I've brought you a drink,' 'I've got a yoghurt for you.' They often check both physically and verbally that the person is comfortable in their bed or chair, with some staff providing a narrative of their actions such as 'I'm just going to sit you up a bit,' 'Let's put another pillow in there.' Despite this apparent communication, it has been shown that during these daily activities staff often fail to spot responses from people with dementia, thereby missing opportunities for communication (Savundranayagam, Sibalija and Scotchmer, 2016). This may be because they are focused more on task completion than on communication. However, for residents these may be the only times when they have one-to-one interactions. It has also been shown that residents who require extra staff effort or higher human resources, such as two staff to move them out of bed, receive fewer care interactions overall (Simmons et al., 2013), thus reducing further their opportunities for communication.

Observation of the communication environment

When we were developing AI we also carried out a more detailed analysis of the communication environment. This involved carrying out an observation of the activity of the person with dementia during the day. We conducted these between 10 a.m. and 3 p.m. using an adapted version of the method of collecting observational data described by Bowie and Mountain (1993) (Table 4.1). Some of the language used in the original measure, devised in 1993, is now outdated. For example, the term 'aimless wandering' is no longer used in dementia care as individuals with dementia are now thought to walk with purpose; hence the new term, 'purposeful walking' was used. We also view the terms 'antisocial' and 'inappropriate' as value-laden terms but during our research we wanted to compare the situation of our participants with that reported by Bowie and Mountain in their 1993 study so we kept these unchanged. Every ten minutes the person with dementia was observed for one minute and a decision made about which category they were engaging in using the modified behaviour categories defined by Bowie and Mountain (1993).

Table 4.1 Observation categories, adapted from Bowie and Mountain (1993)

Category	Description of behaviours
A Self-care	Independent participation in activities of daily living – this includes eating, drinking, dressing, washing and purposeful movement.
B Social engagement	Any activity where the person is appropriately and actively engaged with the environment – this includes participating in social activities, making conversation, reading and watching television.
C Reception of care	Activities where the person is being treated/cared for by staff and is not displaying independence.
D Motor activity	Constant movement and activity – this includes purposeful walking, restlessness, rocking, fidgeting and repetitive movements.
E Antisocial	Behaviours which violate, or cause distress to, others – this includes physical and verbal aggression, screaming or shouting and stealing.
F Inappropriate	Behaviours which would normally be seen as unacceptable, but do not violate others – this includes sucking fingers, urinating inappropriately, spitting or throwing food on the floor and talking to oneself.
G Neutral	Person is detached from the environment – this includes sitting or standing, doing nothing and sleeping.

This observation phase allowed us to collect information that reflected the daily activity and interaction patterns of the people with dementia, thereby providing a picture of their daily routines. Table 4.1 shows the modified behavioural categories and descriptions of those behaviours operationalised by Bowie and Mountain (1993). The descriptions of behaviours in the first three categories (i.e. 'self-care', 'social engagement' and 'reception of care') use adjectives that suggest positive behaviours (i.e. 'independent', 'purposeful', 'appropriately', 'actively', 'cared for') behaviours that might normally be regarded as 'acceptable' or 'typical' of people with dementia in a residential home. Conversely, the remaining four categories ('motor activity', 'antisocial', 'inappropriate', 'neutral') use more negative descriptors (i.e. 'fidgeting', 'violate', 'cause distress', 'aggression', 'unacceptable', 'inappropriately', 'detached'), suggesting behaviours that may appear to be meaningless and/or problematic to caregivers.

In their study, Bowie and Mountain recorded the highest amount of resident time (56.5%) spent in neutral behaviour, 18.75 per cent in motor activity and 8.6 per cent in self-care. Only 0.2 per cent was recorded as antisocial activity. We present the data we collected here to illustrate the social environment of the participants we worked with when we were developing Adaptive Interaction. When the observations of all people with dementia were combined the most common behaviour we recorded was *neutral*, defined by Bowie and Mountain (1993) as the 'person is detached from the environment – this includes sitting or standing and doing nothing and sleeping' (p. 859). This behaviour accounted for 68.65 per cent of the time. Social engagement was only recorded for 10 per cent of the day. There was no antisocial behaviour recorded during the observation period. When compared with the 1993 data recorded by Bowie and Mountain, we can see great similarity. The participants we observed were less physically active – often in bed or a wheelchair – so there was less reported motor activity (2%) and more time assessed as neutral. What became very clear from this observation of the communication environment was the lack of social interaction and opportunities for interpersonal communication that the people with dementia without speech had throughout the period we observed them.

This detailed observation is quite time-consuming and although we found it useful during the process of developing AI, we do not feel it is necessary for successfully using AI. However, to capture important information about the communication environment, we have created a modified version that can be completed with the Getting to Know You chart. This comprises a couple of boxes to fill in for each person with dementia. This will not involve two days of constant observation. Rather, it requires thinking about the person as an individual, who their visitors are and the sort of communication the person might have the opportunity to engage in. An example of a completed Communication Environment chart is provided below in Chart 4.2.

The Communication Environment	
How often do people interact with this person in a typical day?	Hetty spends most of her time in the dayroom in front of the TV. Staff members don't tend to interact with her while she is in the dayroom as she seems contented. Carers chat to Hetty when they get her up and dressed in the morning or when they help her to shower or eat. But she does not respond to them. Her brother Sam comes to visit every second day but he mostly talks to staff members and to residents who can speak.
What 'type' of communication most often occurs? 'Functional' (task-based) or 'social'?	I would say the communication that occurs most often is functional. The carers do chat away to her now and again but they never expect or receive a response from Hetty.

Chart 4.2 Sample Communication Environment chart

Step 3: Identifying the communicative repertoire

The third step of the AI process is identifying the individual's unique repertoire of communication behaviours. These are based on the pre-speech fundamentals of communication outlined in Chapter 3 and include facial expressions, eye gaze and sounds. In identifying the communication repertoire we also look at speech and speech sounds, physical contact, and expression of emotion. Turn-taking, gestures and imitation also form part of the nonverbal communication repertoire. We also record information about the physical position the person is in during an interaction as this helps to understand the options available for communicating. Each category is described briefly below.

Eye gaze

Eye gaze has long been recognised as an important component in nonverbal communication. Back in 1986 Kleinke listed the following functions of eye gaze: 'to provide information, regulate interaction, express intimacy, exercise social control, and facilitate service and task goals' (p. 78). In respect of regulating interactions, recent research using eye tracking technology has shown that eye gaze signals the starting and ending of turns in an interaction (Ho, Foulsham and Kingstone, 2015). This is particularly important when interacting with people who are nonverbal. In our research, we found it useful to distinguish the following types of eye gaze behaviour: eyes open or closed; looking at partner's face or body; looking elsewhere (Ellis and Astell, 2008). However, it is not always possible to tell where someone is looking or if they have their eyes open which is often related to their physical position or posture (see the section 'Body position' below).

Facial expressions

Facial expressions of emotion are universal, that is, they are produced by people of all cultures regardless of language or literacy (Matsumoto and Hwang, 2011). Darwin was the first to put forward this idea as part of his theory of evolution in 1872 and extensive research over the past 145 years has supported his claim. For a long time, it was believed there were six universal facial expressions: joy, sadness, fear, anger, disgust, and surprise, but more recently contempt has been added (Matsumoto and Hwang, 2011). As pointed out in Chapter 2, we can process these facial expressions from birth (Batty and Taylor, 2003). Further evidence of the universality of facial expressions comes from the finding that they occur spontaneously in people who are born blind (e.g. Galati, Miceli and Sini, 2001). We have found that these expressions are retained throughout life and can be seen on the faces of people with dementia who can no longer speak (Ellis and Astell, 2017).

Speech

It may seem strange to include speech when recording information about nonverbal communication. However, we have found that the loss of words is a gradual process and many people retain one or two words for a long period. They may produce these infrequently and at intervals that seem unpredictable. Other people may repeat one single word over and over. The purpose of recording any words is to produce a complete description of an individual's communication repertoire. As explained previously, the aim of AI is not to try to fix the speech of people with dementia. It is to enable their communication partners to connect with them and engage in social interactions. Any speech they make is a part of that process but is not the focus of it.

Sounds

Aside from speech a person's communication repertoire can include a wide variety of sounds. Analysis of spontaneous conversation has shown that approximately half of the speech sounds used in everyday conversation are nonverbal. These are often regarded as 'noise' but these sounds signal important emotional information (Campbell, 2007). Once you start attending to them, the variety of sounds is extensive with many subtle variations. For instance, you may distinguish laughing, chuckling or giggling. Other sounds people make include sighing, coughing, snorting, and breathing heavily. Some people cry out or shriek which can be very loud and attention-grabbing. Others make very subtle, barely discernible sounds. We have also seen people apparently attempting to make sound by moving their mouths and tongues. And some people make no sound at all.

Physical contact

Physical contact is fundamental to human interactions. The quality of physical contact has long been recognised since Harlow (1958) described his studies which found that neonate monkeys preferred a foam rubber and cloth mother over a wire mother, even when the wire mother provided milk and warmth. This study formed part of Harlow's work investigating the basis of love and affection and provided strong support for the importance of contact in their development. While these experiments are now viewed as controversial and it is doubtful such work would receive ethical approval today, the findings in relation to the importance of physical contact have stood the test of time.

More recent research has explored the complexity of touch in human interactions and affiliation, including the role of hormones and neurotransmitters. Touch can be soothing and pleasurable and is often used to convey positive signals such as sympathy, reassurance and comfort (Hertenstein et al., 2006). Evidence for the positive effects of touch has been linked to the release of oxytocin, a neuropeptide that is part of the stress response cycle. Research has linked the plasma oxytocin levels in mothers during pregnancy and the early period after birth with maternal bonding behaviour including eye gaze, high-pitched vocalisations and affectionate touch (Feldman, Singer and Zagoory, 2010). In romantic relationships Holt-Lunstad, Birmingham and Light (2014) found that the quality of the relationship was linked to oxytocin levels in both partners, with happier couples having higher oxytocin levels.

The use of touch with people who have dementia has long been recommended (e.g. Ernst and Shaw, 1980). However, there is also evidence that much of the touch that occurs is during functional tasks, such as providing physical care, and opportunities for more therapeutic or positive touch are lost (Gleeson and Timmins, 2004). To address this, various training programmes and interventions have been developed to equip families and formal caregivers to deliver touch to people with dementia. In describing the communication profile of people with dementia who cannot speak we record any physical contact they make.

Gesture

Gestures are movements that convey information and frequently accompany speech. They occur across cultures and as with facial expressions, gestures have been found in children who are born blind (Iverson and Goldin-Meadow, 1997). Research into the development of gestures and their role in communication has produced different classifications. For example, four categories of gestures have been described in infants under ten months old (Nelson, 1985). These are *expressive gestures*, which are movements used to express emotions (e.g. clapping, tapping feet); *instrumental gestures*, used to control the behaviour of another (e.g. reach out a hand to ask to sit on someone's lap); *enactive gestures*, which are actions with some level of symbolism (e.g. hand beside the face representing sleep); and *deictic* gestures which are used to indicate other objects (e.g. pointing; Lima and Cruz-Santos, 2012). The evolution of these gestures into language occurs through interaction with adults and involves a degree of imitation or mirroring. For example, joint attention occurs when one partner points to an object or person in the environment and looks at their partner (Goldin-Meadow, Mylander and Franklin, 2007). Capturing the gestures of people with dementia without speech is important; these gestures can include pointing, nodding, shaking the head, and many other movements of the hand or body.

Imitation

The importance of imitation in II was introduced in Chapter 3. In our early work developing AI we explored the role of imitation in keeping interactions going in dementia when speech was no longer functional (Astell and Ellis, 2006). Building on the work of Jacqueline Nadel and her colleagues with children with autism spectrum disorders in the early 2000s, we used imitation to make a connection with people with dementia who cannot speak. Nadel et al. (2000) argued that mirroring the actions of individuals with ASD provided them with the opportunity to lead and set the pace of interactions. As we have seen, parents of newborns typically repeat and reinforce the facial expressions, sounds and movements made by their infants. This imitative behaviour forms the basis of their early interactions and provides the foundation for future communication. In parent–infant interactions this reciprocal behaviour arises quite naturally and is both spontaneous and unselfconscious (Tomasello, 1992). In working with people who have dementia and can no longer speak we look for examples of imitation by the individuals with dementia of movements or sounds made by their communication partners.

Body position

As indicated in Chapter 2, body positon and proximity also play important roles in communication. As we saw previously, Burgoon and colleagues (1984) found that leaning forward or in towards your communication partner is an indication of engagement or connection. Mehrabian (1971) also noted the importance of abbreviated movements during an interaction. This includes things such as learning forward in a chair or edging backwards to end a conversation. He pointed out that 'People are drawn toward persons and things they like, evaluate highly, and prefer; and they avoid or move away from things they dislike, evaluate negatively or do not prefer' (Mehrabian, 1971, p. 1).

Posture is also an important indicator of mood. For instance, a drooping or collapsed posture is recognised as an indicator of low mood whereas standing tall with head up is a positive and confident sign. Lhommet and Marsella (2015) synthesised several studies of posture and found that there is strong evidence for identifying emotion from posture. Their analysis included emotions plus pride which was symbolised by 'Head backward or lightly tilted, expanded posture, hands on the hips or raised above the head' (Lhommet and Marsella, 2015, p. 279). In our work, we record the position and posture of the person with dementia who cannot speak during each interaction. Sometimes they are not positioned in the most conducive position for interaction, such as lying in bed facing the wall, but documenting this is important for understanding where and when communication takes place.

Emotion

As we have already learnt, emotion is a composite of multiple nonverbal behaviours including facial expression, posture and gestures. Although these are captured individually, we have found that recording our perceptions of the emotional state of individuals with dementia who cannot speak during an interaction is an important additional feature. Attribution of emotional states of ourselves and others has long been investigated. These judgements require consideration of the context in which emotion occurs and inferences about oneself and others. The term 'psychological distance' has been coined to describe the ways we make judgements about other peoples' emotions (Ong, Goodman and Zaki, 2017). Ong and colleagues (2017) found that humans attribute fewer positive and more negative emotions to people who are dissimilar to them than to ones who are similar. This has important implications for attributing emotions to people with dementia who cannot speak, as we have previously seen that caregivers often distance themselves from the reality of dementia. This reinforces the importance of examining the physical and social environment in which the emotional state of the person with dementia is being judged.

Turn-taking

Turn-taking is another integral part of communication, which effectively regulates interactions between dyads or groups of people. In most communication only one person speaks at a time and the judgement of when another turn is taken is finely tuned such that gaps in speaking are the correct length for another person to speak (Stivers et al., 2009). Research suggests that turn-taking includes anticipation of a response, prediction that another turn will take place, as well as recognition of the end points of turns (Holler et al., 2015). Investigation of language development has shown that at 8–21 weeks, infants are both participants in and initiators of turn-taking sequences (Gratier et al., 2015). It is therefore unsurprising that, as with the other fundamentals of communication, turn-taking appears to be retained in dementia even when speech has gone (Ellis and Astell, 2008). However, the turns and communicative bids of people with dementia who cannot speak may be overlooked by people around them. Therefore, examining 'usual' interactions for signs of turn-taking is vitally important.

PAUSE FOR THOUGHT: NONVERBAL INTERACTION

Now that you have read a description of each of the types of nonverbal behaviour, think of a recent interaction you have had, maybe at home or at work or in a social environment such as shop or coffee bar or on the street. Recreate that interaction in your mind and start to break it down into each of the categories.

Who was the interaction with? Was it a friend or family member, or an employee of an organisation such as a shop assistant, barista or traffic warden?

What was the context? Was it a planned meeting? An unexpected event or a routine, daily interaction?

Was the tone positive, negative or neutral?

Besides speech, did you make any sounds, such as 'uhuh' or 'uhhm'? Did you take turns or did one of you dominate the interaction? Did you nod your head or shrug your shoulders? Did you touch the other person or point to something? Was there any imitation of movements or sounds? Did you smile or frown or pull another face? What about eye gaze – were you looking at them or somewhere else?

How about your posture and position: were you leaning in, standing tall or holding back from them? And how did you feel?

Thinking back through your own interactions should help to confirm the salience of the communication environment in social interactions, as well as the familiarity of nonverbal behaviours in our everyday communication, and how common they are.

As mentioned above, during training we ask caregivers to carry out a usual interaction as a starting point for learning the language of the person with dementia who cannot speak. It might seem strange at first but it is very important for being able to develop a new communication relationship. During AI training, we use video recording to capture these usual interactions.

Once the usual interaction is completed we use the following chart (Chart 4.3) to identify each person's individual communication repertoire. The aim is just to look for each type of behaviour and record if it occurred. We are not interested in amount of times or frequency, just whether the behaviour occurred. See below for an example of a chart completed by a staff member about a person with dementia for whom they care.

Fundamentals of Communication	
1. Eye gaze	Lots of eye contact with me. Narrowed her eyes a lot.
2. Facial expressions	Quite a 'blank' expression but also frowned from time to time.
3. Speech/speech sounds	No speech although we have heard her say 'No' and 'God' before.
4. Sounds	Didn't make any sound today but sometimes she does.
5. Physical contact	I held and stroked her hand. She didn't pull away and seemed to like it.
6. Gestures	Raised her hand and finger as though she was pointing at something. Can't be sure though.
7. Imitation	No imitation that I could see.
8. Bodily position	She was lying on her back and needed me to be standing over her so that she could see me.

9. Emotion	She frowns a lot – maybe she is upset. I didn't see her smile or appear happy.
10. Turn-taking	I didn't see any I don't think.

Chart 4.3 Sample Fundamentals of Communication During 'Usual' Interaction chart

Step 4: Creating a connection

After we have completed the Fundamentals of Communication chart, the next step is to identify one behaviour that can be used as the basis of an interaction. The trainees are encouraged to initiate a new interaction and look for a behaviour they can imitate or reflect to their partner. The aim is to create a connection using a behaviour from the repertoire of the person with dementia. This is the first chance to try using nonverbal means and we encourage trainees to focus their attention onto the individual. To do this, these interactions should take place independently of any other activities. That is, the communication is not taking place during a care activity or a meal or moving around the care setting. In other words, the interaction is the purpose of being together.

Fundamentals of Communication	
1. Eye gaze	Sheila had her eyes open and I tried to copy her blinking but she did not seem to respond.
2. Facial expressions	Sheila's face was neutral most of the time and I did not see anything to pick up on.
3. Speech/speech sounds	Sheila did not say any words.
4. Sounds	Sheila did not make any sounds that I noticed
5. Physical contact	I gently stroked Sheila's arm but she pulled it away.
6. Gestures	After pulling her hand away Sheila looked at me, then at her hand, then she moved her hand towards me. I moved my hand towards hers and she moved her hand again, away from me. I then moved my hand closer to hers and moving our hands became the focus of our interaction.

7. Imitation	I imitated Sheila in moving my hand after she did.
8. Bodily position	I was sitting at 90 degrees to Sheila as she sat in a chair.
9. Emotion	Sheila did not smile or show any specific emotion but she did seem to be concentrating when we were moving our hands.
10. Turn-taking	We took it in turns to move our hands.

Chart 4.4 Sample Fundamentals of Communication chart – creating a connection

Step 5: Building the connection

AI is a holistic approach to communication with an individual that is intended to be used in all interactions. As such our training involves caregivers carrying out multiple interactions with their partner with dementia to build up their connection. We also aim to build confidence in using nonverbal means as the primary form of communication. After focusing on one communication behaviour in the first AI session, we encourage trainees to extend their skills and confidence by picking up on their partner's communication behaviours. The key element is to attend to and imitate their partner's behaviour as the basis of a two-way interaction. For example, if their partner makes a sound, they can imitate it directly or reflect it back in another way, such as tapping or humming. Similarly, if their partner makes small movements, then they could copy or extend them.

Fundamentals of Communication	
1. Eye gaze	Barry's eyes were closed when I approached him but he opened them when I spoke his name. He looked at me and I kept his gaze as I sat beside his chair. His eye contact was very strong and he kept looking at me.
2. Facial expressions	Barry was looking at me and three times during our interaction a small smile came on his face.
3. Speech/speech sounds	Barry does not have any words but as he looked at me he opened his mouth and moved his tongue as if he were trying to speak.

4. Sounds	When Barry was opening his mouth, he made some low sounds that I could just hear if I bent in closer to him.
5. Physical contact	I put out my hand to Barry and he grasped my fingers and held on to them. I offered him my other hand and he held that too and we were squeezing each other's hands.
6. Gestures	As we held hands Barry moved his head a little closer to me when he was trying to speak.
7. Imitation	Both Barry and I leant in towards each other as we held hands and smiled.
8. Bodily position	Barry was facing towards me and we both moved in closer to each other.
9. Emotion	Barry smiled and seemed happy during our interaction.
10. Turn-taking	Barry and I took turns in moving closer to each other and squeezing hands.

Chart 4.5 Sample Fundamentals of Communication chart – building the connection

Summary

AI is an approach that requires practice: first, to overcome embarrassment at using purely nonverbal means to communicate, and second, to allow time to get to know the person with dementia who cannot speak. This process involves multiple interactions as the intention is that AI becomes the channel of communication with people with dementia who are nonverbal. Over time, the communication partners become familiar with the way the individual interacts and the ways in which they respond. They also get to know their variability and differences in mood and situations. They also learn that interactions can vary from day to day even in people with the most minimal of communication behaviours. Becoming intimately familiar with an individual's communication repertoire, their channels of communication – eye gaze, movement, sounds, gestures, the way they move their body towards or away from a person interacting with them – should underpin everyday interactions and enhance recognition of changes in the individual, such as signs of distress, pain or discomfort.

Chapter 5

A Beautiful Noise

Chrissie's Story

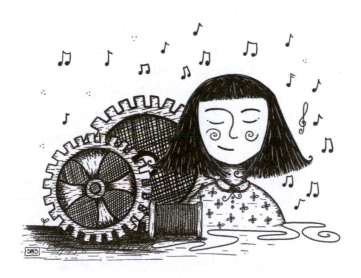

Each of the following three chapters will focus on the individuals with advanced dementia who were introduced to you in Chapter 1. The chapters will begin with a reminder of each person in terms of their history and background and will go on to describe how the trainees worked with the individuals using the AI process.

Chrissie

Chrissie is 78 years old and has been resident in Roseford Care Home for three years. Chrissie appears to be a very happy lady and is known to hum, tap her feet and 'drum' on the side of her chair when music is playing. Chrissie loves to hug and be hugged and will often take people's hands when they sit with her. She more often than not has a smile on her face and often laughs out loud – seemingly for no apparent reason. The care staff are extremely fond of Chrissie but she never seems to engage when they talk to her. Speech doesn't appear to be very meaningful to Chrissie.

Chrissie is unable to walk now and is confined to a wheelchair. Although she loves company, Chrissie spends a lot of time alone in her room, largely because she has a 'signature' sound that she makes – a very high-pitched and loud sound. Other residents and their visitors at Roseford are known to become distressed in response to the sound and staff members find it difficult to carry on with their work when she 'starts'. As such, Chrissie is often taken to her room in her wheelchair at times when she makes the sound and the door is closed on her to prevent other people hearing her.

Chrissie worked in a mill for most of her working life and enjoyed the company of the many friends she made there. A very outgoing and funny woman, Chrissie had a wicked sense of humour and would often play practical jokes on her colleagues and family members. She loved to sing and would take every chance she could to get a sing-song going at parties and get-togethers. Her friends described her as the life and soul of the party and she never turned down a chance to get together with friends and family.

She and her husband Phil had four children and were happily married for 43 years until Phil died suddenly of a massive stroke. Chrissie's family found out very quickly when Phil died just how much he had been doing for Chrissie behind the scenes. Her family had noticed that Chrissie was having some, what they thought to be, minor memory problems but they put that down to her 'getting older'. She was quickly diagnosed with dementia after going outside in her nightdress first thing in the morning. She was found outside the university building where her daughter Jean worked at 6 a.m. The police were called and Chrissie became a resident at Roseford soon after.

Chrissie is visited mostly by her daughter Jean, to whom she has always been very close. Jean always finds her mum to be in high spirits and very tactile and loving when she visits her and she never seems to get upset when Jean has to leave. Despite her largely happy disposition, Chrissie can become very upset during personal care tasks. She is never violent but is known to cry for a long time after she has been taken to the toilet or showered. Neither the care staff nor Jean have any idea why this might be and carers typically dread these types of activities as they know that Chrissie will become extremely distressed. Jean and the staff of Roseford would love to find a way to help Chrissie to stay relaxed during personal care.

Let's now think about what life might be like for Chrissie and how she may view what is going on around her.

CHRISSIE'S PERSPECTIVE

Chrissie is wide awake and alert to what is going on around her. She sees a bustling and confusing environment full of people and different sounds. She hears loud bangs and crashes, people talking and shouting around her, and she can hear music. But it's not music she recognises. It's loud and fast and it thumps but she can hear some people singing along to it. Chrissie sees people walking by her – always in a hurry. She smiles and nods to them but they rarely stop to interact with her. She would love it if someone – anyone – sat down beside her to hold her hand or to give her a hug.

The music in the background is getting louder and louder and Chrissie starts singing to drown it out. She sings at the top of her voice and smiles and laughs as she sees a woman walking towards her. Maybe she wants to join in? The person walking towards her goes directly past her and Chrissie feels her chair start to move. The woman behind her now opens a door and she and Chrissie go inside. The woman leans over Chrissie and says something to her but Chrissie doesn't understand what she said. Another person comes into the room and both strangers start moving Chrissie around and removing her clothes. Chrissie is suddenly terrified as she doesn't understand what is happening to her and why. She cries out in terror and tries to stop them, to no avail. The women place Chrissie in a bed, tuck her in tightly, then leave, closing the door behind them. Chrissie is left upset and alone and cries for what feels like hours.

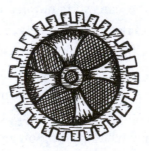

Let's now try to imagine the different feelings that Chrissie might experience throughout the above scenario.

She may feel:

- **ignored** because no-one responds to her when she smiles or joins in when she sings

- **afraid** because she doesn't know what is happening to her when the carers are in her room

- **helpless** because there is nothing she can do to make them stop

- **isolated** because she is left alone in tears.

Stacey

Stacey is the manager at Roseford Care Home and oversees the unit where Chrissie lives. She has been working as a care home manager for 15 years and has often felt that dementia care can be stagnant and that the standard of care has stayed the same since she started. She laments the fact that dementia care is still focused on tasks and that very little is available in the way of maintaining or creating social connection with the residents – especially those at more advanced stages. Having recently undertaken a distance learning course on dementia care, she is aware that there is lots of new and exciting dementia research 'out there'. However, she doesn't see or hear any evidence of the findings of this research being put into practice in the 'real world'. This really frustrates Stacey and she is always looking for something new to try with her residents.

Stacey notices that Chrissie is often in her bedroom even when activities are taking place in the communal lounge. Chrissie also has her meals taken to her room a lot of the time. Stacey is aware that other residents and their families are disturbed by the sounds that Chrissie makes.

STACEY'S PERSPECTIVE

Chrissie seems to be a very contented lady. She has a ready smile and constantly watches what is going on around her. She nods to us as we go about our work and to other residents who walk by her. We sometimes have the radio on at work and it is usually tuned to a station that plays chart music – it keeps the younger carers happy! It seems as though Chrissie tries to sing along to the music as sometimes she starts making this really loud noise. The carers especially can't stand this noise as it's grating and distracting. The other residents tend to get upset by the noise too and it can set everyone off. When she 'starts' we usually use this time to take her to her room for personal care. However, this can be very stressful for Chrissie and the carers as she can get very upset during this time. We usually have to recruit at least two people to help her to go to the toilet or to shower as Chrissie is typically resistant and often cries a lot. We try to comfort her by giving her a hug but she pushes us away. At this point we have no choice but to tuck her up in bed to keep her from harming herself and leave her for a while to calm down.

Let's now think about how Stacey feels in response to the above situation.

She may feel:

- **frustrated** because when Chrissie makes that noise, everyone gets upset – staff, residents and family members

- **helpless** because there is nothing she can do to make her stop

- **sad** because she doesn't want to have to remove Chrissie from the dayroom but she feels she has no choice

- **concerned** because Chrissie gets so upset during personal care and Stacey doesn't know what to do to prevent or deal with this.

PAUSE FOR THOUGHT: THE NURSERY

Try to imagine a situation that may feel very strange to you. You work in a nursery looking after 30-plus babies and young infants. The staff there pay very little attention to the babies because they can't talk so they spend most of their time either talking to each other or interacting

---

with the infants who are learning to speak. When babies cries they are changed or fed then put back in their cot. If they cry again they are left to get on with it – they'll stop eventually. The staff and toddlers chat away and sing together in the playroom while the babies are left alone. This feels really upsetting, doesn't it? It's almost unbearable to even think that this might happen. Usually, if we checked that the baby had everything she needed physically, yet continued to cry, we would most likely pick her up and give her a cuddle. We might also imagine that she could be feeling pain somewhere. The point is that we would investigate, we would be curious. Can we say that this would always be the case when we consider the care provided to people with dementia?

Training in Adaptive Interaction

Stacey recently attended a dementia care conference where she heard about AI: a new approach to communicating with people with advanced dementia. She was fascinated and encouraged by the video clips she saw of the technique in use and was heartened to hear that training in the approach was available. When she went back to Roseford and had a look around it became clear to her that the training would be beneficial to all concerned: first and foremost, the residents with advanced dementia would be afforded re-entry into a world where social interaction is possible, and, second, family members would have the chance to re-engage with their loved ones on some level. Third, Stacey reasoned that her staff and family members of the residents would benefit from learning how to view communication as something that needn't be dependent on the ability to speak. Therefore, as well as improving and expanding their skill set, the staff might change their views on what it is possible to achieve with people with advanced dementia. Furthermore, family members might be able to reconnect with their loved ones from whom they have been isolated for so long. Stacey felt that it was important as manager that she lead by example and become one of the first trainees of AI in Roseford. She was partnered with Chrissie as she knew her well but wanted to know even more about her and to find a way to interact with her. This chapter tells the story of Stacey and Chrissie and of how their relationship blossomed over the course of the training. Along with several others, a relatively new employee, James, and Betty, a friend of one of the residents, also signed up to take part. Chapters 6 and 7 will tell their stories.

Step 1: Getting to know Chrissie

As we saw in Chapter 4, the first stage of the training is to complete the Getting to Know You chart. Stacey had known Chrissie since she came to live at Roseford and so knew bits and pieces about her. In order to find out more, Stacey spent a while chatting and going through the questions on the chart with Chrissie's daughter Jean.

Getting to Know You	
How much personal information do you know about the person, e.g. previous occupation, number of children, hobbies?	Chrissie was employed in a mill for most of her working life. She has four children: Jean, Allison, Rachel and Graham. She has always loved music and continues to enjoy it to this day. She was a very confident and humorous lady.
What do you know about the person's life before he/she became ill?	Chrissie lived at home with her husband. Her difficulties were brought to the fore when he died suddenly. She was quickly admitted to Roseford after a diagnosis of dementia.
What are the person's likes and dislikes?	Chrissie loves music and is a very tactile person. However, she can become very upset when she is receiving personal care.

What are the obstacles to communicating with this person?	Chrissie has one or two words that she uses to communicate but she doesn't seem to understand what is being said to her. She makes a very loud sound that can be disruptive to staff, residents and their family members. We regularly take Chrissie to her room when she starts making 'her' noise. Chrissie also chews her thumb from time to time. Her daughter Jean thinks that this perhaps 'means' that Chrissie is bored but I think it puts people off trying to communicate with her. It just seems so strange to see an adult behaving in this way.
How do you think he/she might be currently feeling and why?	I think Chrissie might be feeling like we ignore her because we don't know how to respond to the sound she makes and will typically remove her from the dayroom if she gets too loud. She may also be angry or afraid because she really doesn't like personal care. This may also lead her to feel helpless because she is at our mercy during personal care. I would say that she will most definitely experience feelings of isolation because we tend to leave her alone to calm down after personal care.
How do you feel when you try to interact with him/her and why?	I get frustrated because when Chrissie makes that noise, everyone gets upset – staff, residents and family members. I also feel helpless because there is nothing I can do to make her stop. This makes me feel sad because I don't want to have to remove Chrissie from the dayroom but I feel I have no choice. I also feel concern because Chrissie gets so upset during personal care and I don't know what to do to prevent or deal with this.

Chart 5.1 Getting to Know Chrissie

We can see from the chart above that Stacey already knows about Chrissie, and has also learned some previously unknown information that might be useful in terms of communicating with her.

Step 2: The communication environment

The second step in the AI process of learning Chrissie's language was to explore her current communication context. This involved using the Communication Environment chart first seen in Chapter 4. Stacey spent a couple of days taking note of who interacted with Chrissie and when. Stacey also paid attention to what sort of communication occurred at these times: whether it was 'functional' or 'social' in nature. It wasn't possible for Stacey to observe Chrissie's situation constantly for two days as she was so busy with the day-to-day running of the home. As such, Stacey took a note of Chrissie's communication environment when Stacey had a spare minute or whenever she witnessed someone interacting with Chrissie. We neither imagine nor recommend that you attempt to observe your communication partner for two days either. Instead, we suggest that you approach this step of the AI process in the same way as Stacey, that is, when you have some spare time or when you observe an interaction.

The Communication Environment	
How often does someone interact with this person in a typical day?	Over the past two days, I have seen five different staff members interacting with Chrissie. Four of them spoke to Chrissie during care tasks, e.g. showering, bathing, eating, etc. and one said 'hello' to Chrissie when she was sat in the day room. Chrissie's daughter visited her mum once over the last two days. She sat with Chrissie in her room and held her hand. Chrissie seemed to enjoy seeing her daughter and smiled a lot while she was there. The noise Chrissie makes was very loud at times when Jean visited.
What 'type' of communication most often occurs? 'Functional' (task-based) or 'social'?	What I have seen over the last two days is that the majority of the communication that is offered to Chrissie is functional in nature. The only real 'social connection' I witnessed was between Chrissie and Jean. They sometimes sort of interact without talking – it's lovely to see but it's not really communication.

Chart 5.2 Chrissie's Communication Environment

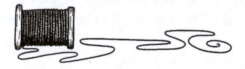

What we read in Stacey's notes above can be summarised in the following main points.

- Chrissie has little opportunity for social communication and most of the interaction she experiences happens during care tasks.

- Chrissie mainly experiences social interaction when her daughter visits.

- Her sound gets louder when her daughter engages with her.

- Stacey doesn't feel that this is 'real' communication.

Step 3: Identifying the communication repertoire

As outlined in Chapter 4, the next step of the AI process is to identify your partner's communication repertoire. This is conducted by engaging in a 'typical' interaction using the Fundamentals of Communication chart to note what occurs in each category. In our training programme, we use video recording to allow group observation and discussion.

As the manager at Roseford, Stacey didn't spend much time involved in hands-on care with the residents and so she wasn't sure what a typical interaction would look like. Therefore, she decided it was best to just go in and talk to Chrissie and see what happened. What took place in the first interaction between Chrissie and Stacey is outlined below.

When Stacey entered her room, Chrissie was lying in her bed, which had padded cot-sides. She was lying on her side on two pillows and her eyes were open. Stacey said 'hello' and Chrissie made 'her' high-pitched sound and fixed her gaze on her. Chrissie continued to make her sound intermittently while looking at Stacey. Chrissie's behaviour in response to Stacey talking to her – making a sound and maintaining direct eye contact – suggested that she wanted to interact.

Very quickly in the interaction (around 30 seconds) Chrissie became silent and she closed her eyes very soon after. Stacey felt that these actions indicated that Chrissie didn't want to continue. However, after a few more seconds Chrissie opened her eyes and with a surprised expression made her high-pitched sound. Stacey continued to talk to Chrissie, passing the time of day by asking her questions such as, 'Have you seen the weather today?' and 'It's not very nice, is it?' Stacey felt that even if Chrissie couldn't answer her verbally, she might be able to nod or shake her head to indicate 'yes' and 'no' if she understood what was being said but she never did. Chrissie kept her gaze fixed on Stacey and at around a minute in, she began chewing her thumb.

This action was one previously identified by Chrissie's daughter as a possible indicator of boredom and may serve as a comfort behaviour for Chrissie (Coia and Jardine Handley, 2008). A few seconds later Chrissie closed her eyes and continued to chew her thumb for a short while. She then removed her thumb from her mouth and her eyes remained closed for the rest of the time Stacey was there. Stacey continued to speak to Chrissie but *she never again opened her eyes, moved or made a sound* during the remainder of the time she was there.

The total interaction lasted for barely one minute of a planned five-minute session. The exchange revealed that although Chrissie appeared to respond to speech at the outset of the session, Stacey's speech alone failed to maintain her participation. This session confirmed the reports from staff of the difficulties they experienced in communicating with Chrissie in regard to basic activities of daily living. However, the session also contained a number of behaviours, such as high-pitched sound and thumb-chewing, that Chrissie's daughter had suggested have a communicative value. These stood out as exactly the sort of behaviours that are used in AI to develop a connection. Below is Stacey's Fundamentals of Communication chart for the interaction just described.

Fundamentals of Communication	
1. Eye gaze	Chrissie made eye contact with me at first and she also looked around the room a bit but she closed her eyes after a few minutes and then kept them closed until I left.
2. Facial expressions	Overall I would say that Chrissie mostly maintained quite a neutral facial expression throughout. However, I'm sure she looked surprised at one point. She didn't seem to smile or frown.
3. Speech/speech sounds	Chrissie didn't use any words throughout the session.
4. Sounds	Chrissie made the familiar high-pitched sound quite a lot to begin with but it died down and stopped completely when she closed her eyes.

5. Physical contact	There was no physical contact between Chrissie and me. One hand was tucked into the bedcovers and she often had the thumb of her other hand in her mouth. It didn't seem as though she wanted me to touch her.
6. Gestures	Chrissie chewed her thumb a couple of times. Her daughter mentioned to me that she thinks this might be a sign of boredom on Chrissie's part. That may well be true as soon after she closed her eyes and went to sleep.
7. Imitation	She did not imitate anything I did.
8. Bodily position	Chrissie was lying on her side facing the window throughout most of the time I was there. However, she buried her head in the blankets when she closed her eyes.
9. Emotion	I did not see Chrissie show any emotion and I have no idea how she was feeling. However, as I said above, her daughter thinks that she chews her thumb when she is bored.
10. Turn-taking	I didn't see any turn-taking when I watched the video but I could be wrong.

Chart 5.3 Chrissie's communication repertoire

If we look at Stacey's chart we can see that she has identified several behaviours of Chrissie's that could be considered communicative. Stacey is now starting to piece together Chrissie's personal communicative repertoire, or 'language'. Furthermore, she is starting to identify patterns of communication in Chrissie and attributing them with some sort of meaning. Perhaps this doesn't seem like a huge achievement at this early stage but it most certainly is. This stage of the AI process is so crucial, not only because we are learning someone's personal language but also because we are starting to view them in a different way. Stacey is now starting to regard Chrissie as a social being, as someone who can and does interact. Perhaps most importantly, Stacey sees Chrissie as someone who *wants* to interact.

Stacey was eager to feed back to her fellow trainees and the trainers as she was excited by what she had witnessed. More than that, she wanted to tell them that she was starting to view Chrissie in a different way – as a social agent. The training session involved everyone chatting about their experiences and looking at and reviewing each other's videos. The trainees agreed that it was difficult at first to identify communicative actions in their communication partners as they were so used to the idea of communication being all about speech. Watching the videos together allowed them to comment on the interactions and to pick up on behaviours that may not have been clear in the moment. The trainees were asked to identify one action used by their partner that they felt may be of some communicative significance and to try to reflect that to the person during their next interaction. Stacey thought that perhaps the most significant action for Chrissie was her sound. However, Stacey also shared with the group that she would feel awkward and embarrassed while trying to reproduce Chrissie's sound. Perhaps Chrissie would be offended. Perhaps her colleagues would think she'd 'lost it'. Maybe she would fail to connect with Chrissie. As mentioned in previous chapters, these feelings are common in new trainees and it's quite normal to feel this way at first. The trainer discussed these feelings with the group, giving examples from everyday life of when we engage in similar things without even thinking about them.

Step 4: Creating a connection

As you now know, step 4 of the Adaptive Interaction process involves creating a connection with your interaction partner by identifying and reflecting back to them one of their own behaviours or language elements within an interaction (Caldwell, 2005; Caldwell and Horwood, 2007). Furthermore, as illustrated in Stacey's example above, this first foray into reflecting your partner's actions back to them can feel a little strange at first. Nevertheless, feeling bolstered by the trainer's advice and her fellow trainees' encouragement, Stacey gave it her best shot.

Stacey entered Chrissie's room with some trepidation. However, the nervous feeling was soon replaced by sorrow when she saw her communication partner. Chrissie was lying in bed tucked under her blankets, staring out of the window. Stacey felt sad that Chrissie was alone again – she looked so bored! Stacey pulled a chair over to Chrissie's bedside and sat down close by her. As soon as she saw Stacey, Chrissie made eye contact with her and made her sound. Stacey reciprocated by trying to echo Chrissie's sound. Stacey thought she could almost see a smile spread across Chrissie's face, but she wasn't sure. Chrissie's gaze was fixed on Stacey and she continued to do so as she lifted her thumb to her mouth to chew on it. Stacey did the same and Chrissie made a very soft and low sound while holding Stacey's gaze. The pair carried on like this for a few seconds until Chrissie removed her thumb from her mouth and made her sound. Stacey followed suit and the communication partners took turns making the sound for around ten seconds. Chrissie then put her thumb back in her mouth and she and Stacey did this for another few seconds.

Then something different happened. Chrissie circled her lips with her thumb, all the while staring into Stacey's eyes. Chrissie watched Stacey do the same, chewed on her thumb for another couple of seconds then broke her gaze from Stacey, looking down onto the blankets. This surprised Stacey as Chrissie had seemed to be really engaged with her. After a few seconds, Stacey felt she had to do something to keep the interaction going and made Chrissie's sound again. Chrissie raised her eyebrows and quickly shifted her gaze to Stacey and made her sound too, followed by a laugh! This was starting to feel like a game and the little element of surprise (reintroducing Chrissie's sound) introduced by Stacey had made it interesting again for Chrissie. Stacey had never imagined that something so small and seemingly insignificant could make her so proud and happy!

The two continued to take turns using Chrissie's sound – sometimes loud, sometimes soft. They held each other's gaze all the while, then Chrissie looked back down at the bed and fell silent again, this time burying her face in the blankets. Remembering what happened in this situation the last time, Stacey reintroduced the signature sound and Chrissie lifted her head, looked right at Stacey and made her sound again. It felt wonderful but strange to Stacey as it seemed almost like a game of peek-a-boo that you might play with an infant. Should she be engaging in this with Chrissie – a grown woman? Was it age appropriate? It struck Stacey that Chrissie was the lead partner in this interaction and as such had the power to stop or continue as she pleased. If this provided a fun way for the two of them to connect then maybe age appropriateness isn't always…appropriate? The two continued to turn-take with the sound; this time Chrissie was looking back down at the bed. She then put her thumb back in her mouth and when Stacey did the same, Chrissie made eye contact with her again. Turn-taking again took place, this time with a new combination of thumb-chewing and sounds. Chrissie began to get quieter and closed her eyes. She snuggled into the blankets and Stacey thought she had fallen asleep. This time it was Chrissie who surprised Stacey! Chrissie quickly opened her eyes and loudly made her sound, making Stacey laugh. The two of them continued in different combinations of eye gaze, thumb-chewing and sound until Chrissie eventually did fall asleep, effectively ending the session.

Fundamentals of Communication	
1. Eye gaze	Lots of eye contact with me this time. Chrissie also looked down at the bed at several points but always retuned her gaze to me.
2. Facial expressions	I'm pretty sure that Chrissie smiled at me at one point. I think she also looked surprised on a couple of occasions.
3. Speech/speech sounds	I didn't hear any speech from Chrissie.

4. Sounds	Chrissie made 'her' sound a lot during the session. It was very varied in volume. Sometimes it was very loud and uproarious, at other times it was soft and quite soothing.
5. Physical contact	There was no physical contact between myself and Chrissie.
6. Gestures	Chrissie chewed her thumb at several points throughout. I'm starting to think that this isn't a sign of boredom as suggested by her daughter. It seems like it might be another part of her language that she uses to engage with other people. She also introduced a 'new' gesture that I'd never seen her engage in before – circling her lips with her thumb.
7. Imitation	Chrissie did imitate me in this session – I could hardly believe it! At times when she fell silent, I would wait a few seconds and reintroduce her sound. She responded to this by looking at me and making her sound towards me.
8. Bodily position	Chrissie stayed in a similar position throughout the session. She was on her side and would sometimes move her hand underneath the blankets to bring her thumb to her mouth.
9. Emotion	I think I saw Chrissie smile at one point. She also looked surprised on several occasions when I reintroduced her sound. In general I would say that she seemed to be quite excited and buoyed by the interaction. She certainly never seemed to be unhappy or upset.
10. Turn-taking	There was lots of turn-taking this time! We largely took turns using her sound and thumb-chewing. I think I was starting to get better at timing the turns so that I wasn't overlapping with her too much.

Chart 5.4 Connecting with Chrissie

As we can see in Chart 5.4, Stacey was really growing in confidence as the session went on. She started to recognise communicative behaviours in Chrissie in a way that she hadn't before. She also started to change her view of one of Chrissie's behaviours – her thumb-chewing. Stacey's initial trepidation about the AI process was turning into feelings of surprise, curiosity and accomplishment. She was eager to keep practising with Chrissie and to see how far they could get together. Stacey was well aware that Chrissie would never again hold a conversation using speech. But she didn't have to – she had her *own* language. All Stacey had to do was learn it.

Step 5: Building the connection

By the time the group had reached the last week of training, the trainees had lots of practice of engaging in AI with their communication partners. The trainees were now engaging in longer sessions with their partners, constantly building both their skills and confidence. What follows is a description of one of the final interactions between Stacey and Chrissie that took place during training.

Stacey allowed ten minutes to go into Chrissie's room to conduct a session where she attended to and imitated Chrissie's verbal and nonverbal behaviours. For example, if Chrissie made a vocalisation, Stacey may have attempted to imitate it directly or to reproduce the rhythm of it in some way, for example by tapping it out on the side of the bed. As such, Stacey focused on continuing to learn Chrissie's communicative repertoire and reflecting it back to her in a way that was potentially meaningful to her.

At the start of this session Chrissie was lying in her bed with the padded cot-sides. She was lying on her side on two pillows dozing. After a few seconds Chrissie opened her eyes and looked directly at Stacey and made 'her' sound in a high-pitched tone. Stacey immediately reflected the sound and pitch back to her. Chrissie then repeated the sound and they took another two turns each in this manner. As in the previous session, Chrissie's immediate reaction to Stacey speaking was to look at her and make the high-pitched sound. In this session, however, rather than continuing to speak, Stacey adapted her response to match Chrissie's, which resulted in a brief initial 'dialogue' of several turns each.

About half a minute into the interaction, the dialogue changed when Chrissie put her thumb in her mouth and started chewing and chewing on it, all the time looking into Stacey's eyes. Stacey responded by chewing and chewing her own thumb. Chrissie then removed her thumb from her mouth and made her high-pitched sound. Stacey responded by taking her thumb from her mouth and repeating the sound made by Chrissie. Chrissie then put her thumb back into her mouth, and Stacey followed suit. In these exchanges Chrissie took the lead by introducing a new behaviour (thumb-chewing), then reverting to the previous behaviour (high-pitched sound), then returning to thumb-chewing, all the while looking intently at Stacey. Stacey responded to each of these changes by matching Chrissie's behaviour.

Stacey then attempted to change the dialogue by removing her thumb from her mouth and making a sound like Chrissie's high-pitched one. In response Chrissie then removed her thumb from her mouth and matched the sound, and she and Stacey then continued to turn-take making this sound for around another 20 seconds. This section of dialogue ended when Chrissie began chewing her thumb again. In this exchange, Stacey reintroduced one of Chrissie's behaviours (high-pitched sound) and Chrissie responded by altering her own behaviour to match Stacey's.

At around a minute and a half into the session, Stacey attempted to change the interaction again by introducing a new element. This was to imitate the rhythm of Chrissie's thumb-chewing through tapping her fingers on the side of the bed. Chrissie continued to chew her thumb and stared intently at her. After a few seconds, Chrissie removed her thumb from her mouth and made her high-pitched sound. Stacey stopped tapping and repeated the vocal sound and turn-taking resumed using Chrissie's sound until Stacey tapped on the bed again. Chrissie became silent, put her thumb back in her mouth and watched Stacey's fingers tapping on the bed. She then removed her thumb from her mouth and resumed her high-pitched sound. At around two minutes in, Chrissie put her thumb in her mouth and immediately removed it when she saw Stacey do the same. Chrissie and Stacey then resumed turn-taking with her sound.

In this phase, when Stacey introduced the new element (rhythmic tapping) there was no discernible change in Chrissie's behaviour. She continued to chew her thumb while looking intently at Stacey. However, as Stacey continued to tap, Chrissie then stopped chewing and made her high-pitched sound. She did not put her thumb in her mouth again during this session. The turns in this exchange suggest that the introduction of a variation of one her behaviours (thumb-chewing) had less impact for Chrissie than the matched behaviour. However, she appeared to retain her interest in the interaction as she continued to look at Stacey and finally reintroduced a previous behaviour (high-pitched sound).

Chrissie and Stacey continued the dialogue making the high-pitched sound until around two and a half minutes into the interaction, at which point Chrissie introduced another new behaviour. She lifted her head up from the pillows and moved towards Stacey's hand, which was resting on the cot-side. Chrissie rubbed her forehead on Stacey's hand and Stacey responded by stroking Chrissie's hair. Stacey then attempted to reintroduce one of Chrissie's previous behaviours – her thumb-chewing and the rhythm of it. Again, Chrissie raised her head, rubbed her forehead against Stacey's hand and then closed her eyes. Stacey then made Chrissie's sound, to which she reciprocated, followed by a number of turns each. Chrissie continued to keep her eyes closed for almost a minute during this part of the interaction.

This phase of the session was notable for Chrissie introducing touch into the interaction. The dialogue had been proceeding through sound and vision (eye contact) when Chrissie opened up a third channel of communication: touch. However, although Stacey responded by touching Chrissie's head, Stacey did not match her behaviour as she had done with Chrissie's sound.

Stacey felt a bit apprehensive about touching Chrissie as she wasn't sure it was appropriate.

After the sound turn-taking, Chrissie then rubbed her head against Stacey's hand for a third time. It seemed clear to Stacey that Chrissie wanted to connect with her via touch. As such, Stacey moved forward and rubbed her head against Chrissie's. At this point, Chrissie opened her eyes and gave a look of surprise followed by the high-pitched sound. The dialogue then took on the form of a spontaneous game of mutual head touching and vocalisation. During this phase Chrissie laughed at several points after she and Stacey touched heads. This is perhaps the most exciting part of the interaction as this is when Chrissie exerted the most control over the situation and was the most animated. Chrissie was clearly attempting to get closer to and to touch Stacey. However, initially Stacey failed to detect this and was focused on maintaining previous strategies of the interaction. Once Stacey recognised Chrissie's new direction, the interaction took on a new dynamic. From the moment Stacey touched heads with Chrissie, their communication became much more playful. They took turns with sounds and touching and both laughed at several points throughout. Stacey felt that she and Chrissie really connected at this point in the interaction. They were smiling, laughing and were close both physically and emotionally. It felt wonderful!

At around seven minutes into the interaction, Chrissie fell silent and closed her eyes. She remained like this until Stacey touched her head a while later, at which point she made her sound and then opened her eyes when Stacey reciprocated with the sound. Chrissie and Stacey began turn-taking again using Chrissie's sound and both laughed several times. At approximately nine minutes into the interaction Chrissie fell silent and then closed her eyes a few seconds later. This suggested to Stacey that perhaps Chrissie was ready to end the interaction at a point before Stacey realised. Stacey attempted to keep the interaction going and Chrissie reciprocated with enthusiasm for a while but closed her eyes again very soon after. Chrissie closing her eyes effectively ended the interaction and can be seen as another element of her communication repertoire. Chart 5.5 gives Stacey's Fundamentals of Communication chart for the interaction.

Fundamentals of Communication	
1. Eye gaze	Chrissie fixed her gaze on me almost throughout the entire interaction.
2. Facial expressions	Chrissie smiled a lot during the interaction. She also looked surprised a few times.
3. Speech/speech sounds	There was no speech that I could hear.
4. Sounds	There was lots of Chrissie's sound – again, varying in volume and getting louder as touch was introduced.
5. Physical contact	There was a lot of physical contact between myself and Chrissie this time! It took me a while to realise that it was what she wanted and for me to feel comfortable about engaging in it with her.
6. Gestures	Chrissie chewed her thumb at times but the most significant thing I think was her moving her head towards my hand and rubbing against it. This indicated to me that she wanted to engage in touch.
7. Imitation	Chrissie imitated me a lot in this session – she copied sounds, laughing, smiling, touch – so many things!
8. Bodily position	Chrissie was on her side to begin with but moved her body upwards several times so that we could rub heads.
9. Emotion	I don't think I've ever seen Chrissie look so happy! She seemed to be delighted throughout.
10. Turn-taking	Lots of turn-taking again, more than last time I think. We took turns using her sound, touch, smiles and laughter.

Chart 5.5 Building the connection with Chrissie

Group discussion

The trainees and trainer had a final group discussion on the last day of training. They spoke about how they felt the course had gone, and their feelings towards the training. What follows is Stacey's part of the discussion.

Trainer: So Stacey, how do you feel the training has gone?

Stacey: I feel I have really achieved something personally and as a team here at Roseford.

Trainer: OK, great. Can you explain?

Stacey: Yeah – on a personal level, I now think about communication in a different way than I did previously. I recognise that nonverbal communication is just as, if not more important than speech. Especially to people with dementia. I've learned that people with advanced dementia always have the potential to communicate – we just have to find out how to speak each individual's language. I think as a team, we have changed our outlook and expectations and those are huge achievements.

Trainer: That's great. Did you find it difficult to do that?

Stacey: To begin with, yes. But, to be honest it was more about how I felt about doing it than the actual technique itself. I was a bit embarrassed and unsure about the whole thing to begin with and I wondered if it might be demeaning for people with dementia to engage in this sort of communication. However, once I felt I had connected with Chrissie I didn't feel or think those things any more. We really 'got on' and we didn't utter a word to each other!

Trainer: That's excellent – well done! Did you at any point feel that it wasn't working?

Stacey: A couple of times I did wonder if I was doing it right. Some sessions felt more 'successful' than others. In those sessions, Chrissie and I would engage in lots of different behaviours together and I could spend ages writing about it on the 'fundamentals' sheet. At other times, Chrissie was quieter and we didn't do so much together and I struggled to find things to write about. During those sessions I felt compelled to try things that had provoked a response from Chrissie on previous days – just to get a reaction.

Trainer: That's a really important point, Stacey. How did you get over those feelings?

Stacey: I reminded myself of the title of the approach – *Adaptive* Interaction. We have to adapt to our communication partner and how they are on any given day. Just like anyone else, people with dementia can feel low or tired or maybe just want to be left alone. The next day they could be in a great mood and eager to interact. Therefore, it's really important that we go with the flow.

Trainer: What will you change about Chrissie's care now that you have learned about Adaptive Interaction?

Stacey: I think we could start using Adaptive Interaction with her when she is in the dayroom. We might well see changes in how she uses her sound. We could also start playing music that she likes when she is there as Jean says this relaxes her. Perhaps most importantly, we will use Adaptive Interaction with Chrissie when we are delivering her personal care to make her feel safe and that someone is listening to her.

Trainer: Excellent! What do you think is the most important thing you've learned?

Stacey: I would say the most important thing is that the nonverbal stuff *is* actually communication. When I saw Chrissie and her daughter holding hands and laughing together I didn't think it was. But it *is* communication – more important than that, it's *connection*.

Summary

Chrissie's story has shown us that she was crying out – literally – for human interaction. She was ignored and shut away because of this 'terrible' noise she made. The 'terrible' noise was nothing more than a request for a hug or a smile. The caregivers at Roseford can now 'turn the volume down' on Chrissie's sound by reflecting it back to her, making it quieter each time. She usually imitates this and the sound goes from a roar to a whisper. This means that Chrissie gets to stay in the dayroom where the music played is now more appropriate to her generation than it was previously. Chrissie hums along – not always following the tune – but this is *her* language after all.

Chapter 6

I'm Looking Through You

Eleanor's Story

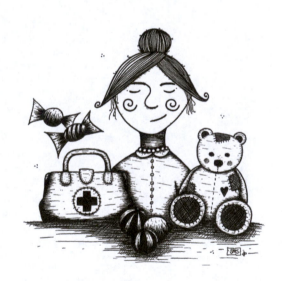

Eleanor

Eleanor is 66 years old and has been living in Roseford Care Home for seven years. She was diagnosed with early onset dementia when she was 55 years old. Eleanor has one daughter, Angie, to whom she is very close. She is also married to Mike – a very supportive man who is clearly devoted to her and her wellbeing.

Eleanor was a children's nurse and the first signs of dementia were when she began to make mistakes at work. The usually self-confident children's nurse became more and more unsure and withdrawn. She would typically attempt to cover up mistakes with a joke and a laugh, never for a minute acknowledging that anything was wrong. At other times, Eleanor would blame her colleagues for her mistakes in a desperate attempt to save face. This upset her work mates and they began to detach themselves from her whenever possible. Eleanor had started avoiding nights out with the girls and stopped gathering with her colleagues at coffee breaks. She was embarrassed by what was happening to her and she wanted to maintain her status and friendships but it became too much to manage. It all came to a head when Eleanor's daughter Angie returned from her gap year and noticed a marked change in her mum's demeanour. She was forgetting appointments, getting lost in the middle of sentences, and had even wet herself when they were out shopping. Angie made an appointment for her mum with the GP and accompanied her. Not long after this, Eleanor was diagnosed with early onset dementia.

Eleven years later Eleanor no longer speaks and doesn't seem to communicate at all. She has a steely look that she appears to reserve for those she doesn't seem to like very much. However, this can change in that one day it might be the doctor, the next day the cleaner or a visiting neighbour – no-one can be sure when she might be feeling this way. The care staff tend to avoid

Eleanor if they can as they find her behaviour unpredictable and hostile, especially during personal care, when she can become very upset. At these times, she can hit out and push them away when they come to assist her to go to the toilet or have a shower. Neither the care staff nor her family have any idea why this might be and care staff typically dread these types of activities as they know that Eleanor will become extremely distressed.

Eleanor is extremely fortunate in terms of her family's commitment to her as she has regular visits from her family and is hardly ever alone. Mike describes himself as her husband, not her 'carer' and is quick to correct anyone who fails to make this distinction. He feels that Eleanor is no longer the person she once was and often fears that he has lost her forever. However, he is willing to explore the possibility that they might be able to reconnect with Eleanor in some way.

Let's now think about what life might be like for Eleanor and how she may view what is going on around her.

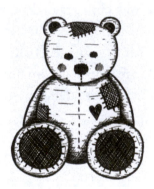

ELEANOR'S PERSPECTIVE

Eleanor feels uncomfortable. She is stuck in bed and is sore all over. She finds it hard to see and to hear what is going on around her and peers into the distance to see what or who is there. She can see shapes and hear sounds but can't make them out. She can only move a little before the pains in her body start off again. She doesn't know where she is and doesn't recognise any of the things she sees or hears. It's as though she isn't really there. Things 'happen' to her body – she is moved around and shifted here and there. Eleanor doesn't understand this and she tries her best to stop it from happening. She longs for something, anything to make sense to her and cries in desperation.

Let's now try to imagine the different feelings that Eleanor might experience throughout the above scenario.

She may feel:

- **fear** because she doesn't know where she is or what is happening around her

- **anger** because she has so many questions about her situation but can't form the words or even fully form her thoughts

- **isolation** because she longs for company and to make sense of the world

- **concern** owing to the physical pain she is experiencing.

James

James is 23 years old and has only been working at Roseford for a couple of months. He has never worked in a care environment before and is still quite nervous. He is finding it hard to acclimatise to his new role and sometimes finds it difficult to know what to do in certain situations. Nevertheless, he is committed to doing a good job and is keen to learn.

JAMES' PERSPECTIVE
Eleanor seems to be unhappy all the time. James has never seen her smile and she frowns a lot. She screws up her face and is known to

glare at people who come into her room. The staff are quite scared of Eleanor as she lashes out during personal care and she has hurt a few of the carers. When James first came to work at Roseford, he was warned about Eleanor and advised to 'get in and get out quickly'. The first time he did this, leaving Eleanor in her room, he could hear her crying as he walked away along the corridor.

Let's now think about how James feels in response to the above situation.

He may feel:

- **apprehension** because colleagues have warned him about Eleanor's behaviour

- **fear** because Eleanor hits out at him when he helps her to change her clothes

- **confusion** because he doesn't understand why Eleanor behaves this way

- **helplessness** because he doesn't know how best to approach Eleanor or to make her feel safe.

PAUSE FOR THOUGHT: A NEW COLLEAGUE

Try to imagine now that a new position has been filled at your place of work. You've been on holiday for the last couple of weeks and haven't actually met your new colleague yet but you are feeling anxious about doing so. While you've been away your friends at work have been texting you, telling you what this new colleague, Holly, is like. They don't seem to be impressed with her and have been complaining to you that she's quiet and moody and doesn't join them for their usual coffee break. They find her to be aloof and don't think she'll fit in. On your return to work, you go in early to give yourself a head start to the day. You find Holly, your new colleague, already working at her desk.

What do you think? If you go with what your friends told you about her, you might think that she came in early to avoid her work mates. She is, after all, unfriendly. However, when you take Holly at face value you find that she is a perfectly pleasant woman who confides in you that she is having trouble adjusting to her new role. You also realise that she is extremely shy and nervous of joining groups. You now begin to understand why your colleagues might have formed such a negative opinion of Holly. They completely misunderstood her.

Training in Adaptive Interaction

Mike and Angie wanted Eleanor to be part of the AI training that was taking place at Roseford as they were informed that the approach might provide a means of communicating with her. James is to be Eleanor's communication partner as he had been working with her a lot recently. He is eager to learn and sees the AI training as a means of expanding his skill set.

Step 1: Getting to know Eleanor

When James started the training with Betty and Stacey, he felt a little apprehensive. He wasn't sure that AI would 'work' for Eleanor as she could often appear to be so hostile. Nevertheless, he felt excited by the prospect of learning something new, a skill that would help him to better connect with the individuals he cares for. The first training activity that James took part in was the Getting to Know You chart. He realised that he knew very little about Eleanor and decided to talk it through with Mike and Angie the next time they visited (Chart 6.1).

Getting to Know You	
How much personal information do you know about the person, e.g. previous occupation, number of children, hobbies?	Eleanor is married to Mike and has one daughter called Angie. Eleanor was a children's nurse in quite a senior position. She was popular with her colleagues and had a wide circle of friends. She enjoyed going out with her friends and was famous for her shopping habit!
What do you know about the person's life before he/she became ill?	Eleanor started having problems at work which highlighted that something was wrong. She went downhill very quickly after diagnosis and now doesn't talk at all and can't move around by herself.
What are the person's likes and dislikes?	Eleanor loves her food and is always keen to eat when food is offered. She loves sweets in particular! Mike keeps a stock of chocolates in her room and they eat them together while he chats to her. It's nice to see.
What are the obstacles to communicating with this person?	It's really hard to even begin communicating with Eleanor because she looks so angry all the time. She hits out and cries when we deliver personal care and I find her quite intimidating.

Chart 6.1 Getting to Know Eleanor

We can see from James' notes that he finds it really difficult to interact with Eleanor. However, he had already made up his mind about her to some extent before he met her due to his colleagues' comments and warnings.

Step 2: The communication environment

The second step in the AI process was for James to explore Eleanor's opportunities for social interaction using the 'Communication Environment' chart. James spent a couple of days observing when someone interacted with Eleanor, who it was and what sort of communication he witnessed. To allow James and the other trainees to do this, James had set aside some protected time for them to take notes at the end of their shift. Below is James' assessment of Eleanor's communication environment (Chart 6.2).

The Communication Environment	
How often does someone interact with this person in a typical day?	I have witnessed around seven members of staff talking to Eleanor over the last two days. Most of these interactions occurred during care tasks. Around three people go in to see her at any given time as she can lash out. One person sang as she took Eleanor to the dining room in her wheelchair but I don't think she was singing to Eleanor per se. Mike visited Eleanor twice over the last two days. He talked to her and held her hand.
What 'type' of communication most often occurs? 'Functional' (task-based) or 'social'?	Most of the communication that I saw taking place was functional. Staff members typically tend to Eleanor as quickly as possible as her manner and actions can be frightening. Mike doesn't have this experience of Eleanor and is always happy to see her. I saw him stroke her hair and feed her chocolates. She didn't smile but seemed more content than usual. I don't know if I would call this a social interaction as it all seemed to be coming from Mike.

Chart 6.2 Eleanor's Communication Environment

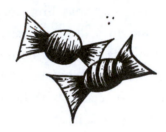

As we can see in the chart James completed, a relatively large number of people interacted with Eleanor over the two-day period: around seven care staff and one family member. However, what is clear is that staff members tend to go into Eleanor's room 'mob-handed', more than likely in anticipation of some sort of violent episode on her part. They do not stay long and keep their interactions to a minimum. Mike and Eleanor have a far more relaxed time together. The pace is slower and although James isn't sure he would call this social interaction, he is aware that it is far more pleasant for Eleanor.

Step 3: Identifying the communication repertoire

The next step James took in the AI training was to identify Eleanor's communication repertoire. This is conducted by engaging in a 'usual' interaction with the person with dementia using the Fundamentals of Communication chart to note what occurs in each category. James was a bit concerned about how he would go about interacting with Eleanor in a 'typical' session as everything he had observed so far was rapid, functional and did not have a social element. In his brief experience of caring for Eleanor, he and his colleagues would go in and out as quickly as possible, with no time spent just in social interaction.

James always felt uncomfortable about the way people interacted with Eleanor and wanted to learn how to approach her instead of avoiding her. After some thought, James decided to take a magazine with him so that they would have something to look at together. Mike had told him about Eleanor's love of shopping and he thought a fashion magazine might spark some interest. What took place in the first interaction between Eleanor and James is outlined below (see Chart 6.3).

Eleanor was sitting up in a chair with her eyes closed. James wished her good morning in a loud voice, attempting to get her to open her eyes, but she didn't stir. He tapped her lightly on the shoulder and said her name again. Eleanor made some movements with her mouth but still didn't open her eyes. There was a lot of noise: buzzers were going off, other carers were chatting nearby and the radio was on. James tried again to get Eleanor's attention by gently touching her chin. She immediately screwed up her face but still didn't open her eyes. James wondered if he would ever get a reaction from Eleanor – she didn't seem to be doing *anything*. He said her name one more time and she half opened her eyes, looked downwards, and then quickly closed her eyes again. James reached for the magazine. He felt that he was floundering and needed something to get them going. James started flicking through the magazine pointing out different celebrities and fashion features. At one point Eleanor rapidly opened her eyes, glared at him, and then closed her eyes again.

James continued to flick through the magazine, talking about what he could see on the pages, but Eleanor continued to keep her eyes closed. James felt like he wasn't making any headway with the magazine and put it down on the table. He gently touched Eleanor's forearm and asked her if she'd had a visit from Mike today. Nothing. 'Have they made your bed today?' Nothing. 'What's for lunch?' Still nothing. This pattern continued for the rest of the time James was with Eleanor. James asked Eleanor a question, she occasionally opened her eyes then quickly closed them again. James felt discouraged. He had hoped he might be able to get some sort of a reaction from Eleanor – something other than closed eyes.

The above interaction between James and Eleanor illustrates James' eagerness to find a method of reaching Eleanor that would encourage her to respond. James tried several different ways of interacting with Eleanor, none of which seemed to 'work', but these were mostly relying on speech, particularly asking her questions. She remained quiet and stony-faced throughout. It seemed he needed to keep talking to Eleanor to fill the silences. He had hoped that showing her the magazine might elicit some sort of response but Eleanor rarely opened her eyes, let alone looked at it. He also touched Eleanor a few times to try to catch her attention. However, James noted that these attempts were either ignored or met with a glower. Below is the chart James completed describing the fundamentals of communication in this interaction.

Fundamentals of Communication	
1. Eye gaze	Eleanor kept her eyes closed for most of the session. She would occasionally open them and either look off to the other side of the room or glare at me.
2. Facial expressions	I found it difficult to identify facial expressions in Eleanor but I think her expression was largely neutral. However, she did screw her face up after I touched her and she seemed to glare at me a couple of times.
3. Speech/speech sounds	No speech.
4. Sounds	No sounds either – she was extremely quiet.
5. Physical contact	I tried to start an interaction using touch a couple of times but other than that there was no physical contact.
6. Gestures	I didn't notice any gestures.
7. Imitation	Eleanor didn't imitate anything I did.
8. Bodily position	She was sitting in a chair and I was at her left side. She was facing forwards.
9. Emotion	The only emotion I could pick up was anger or annoyance. I didn't feel she wanted me there.
10. Turn-taking	I didn't feel that there was any turn-taking between us.

Chart 6.3 Eleanor's communication repertoire

Looking at James' chart for the first interaction between him and Eleanor, it's easy to see why he might be feeling deflated. He found it hard to identify anything in Eleanor's behaviour that he recognised as communication. He also felt that she didn't want to communicate with him at all. James wasn't looking forward to the training feedback session with his peers as he felt he hadn't achieved anything with Eleanor. When he and the rest of the trainees met with the trainers James was not keen to say how it had gone with Eleanor. Stacey and Betty and the other trainees seemed to have made some progress with their communication partners and James felt as though his efforts had gone to waste. Worse still, he felt that he was a failure as he had not made any connection with Eleanor.

The group watched James' video together as he cringed his way through it. However, at the end of the video James' colleagues and the trainers were more positive about the interaction they had just witnessed than he was. Although Eleanor's eyes were closed for most of the session, they pointed out that she did open them at several points, one time when he said her name. This was very brief but she did make a response. The group also noted that Eleanor was making a lot of movements with her mouth and suggested that these might be something that he could work with the next time. One of the other trainees noted that perhaps the reason why Eleanor didn't seem to like it when James touched her is because it came as a shock. Her eyes were closed when he touched so she was not able to anticipate it. The trainer suggested that perhaps touch might be a better way forward when Eleanor's eyes were open.

The final point that the trainer made about the interaction was that Eleanor did not seem to like it when James was talking to her about what he could see in the magazine. She briefly opened her eyes a couple of times and glared at James. They discussed whether she maybe did not like the sound of the talking or that perhaps she could not hear him properly as there was certainly a lot of background noise. Alternatively, they suggested it might simply be because she was trying to sleep. There could be many reasons, but the group suggested that James should wait until Eleanor was wide awake before trying to interact with her.

Afterwards, James spoke briefly to Eleanor's husband, Mike, about how he felt the session had gone. Mike was not in the least bit disappointed. He knew it would not be easy for James to develop a connection with Eleanor as he had seen that the staff found it difficult to interact with her. He was sad that they found Eleanor intimidating and he knew that they avoided her whenever possible. Therefore, he was really pleased that someone other than himself or Angie was attempting to interact with Eleanor purely for the sake of it.

Step 4: Creating a connection

The next morning, James was keen to have another interaction with Eleanor to try some of the things that had been suggested at the group sessions. After seeing how Stacey and Betty and the other trainees had got on, he felt much better about his first interaction with Eleanor. Before the group session, he had assumed that everyone else had interacted with their partners and he was the failure. However, once he saw the other videos he realised that this first step was about understanding what types of interaction the people with dementia were having. He saw that other trainees spoke to their partners and, just as he had, several of them had taken things along to show their interaction partner.

What he had enjoyed most about the group discussion and reflection was paying attention to the ways each person with dementia behaved. James found it fascinating to see the differences between them, but also difference in the ways the other trainees behaved. He wanted to have another try with Eleanor and hoped there would be an opportunity to try reflecting the movement she made with her mouth.

When he approached Eleanor, James made sure that she was sitting comfortably in her wheelchair and then told her he would like to wheel her into a quiet room. He decided to do this because during the session the previous day, when they watched the video, he had been shocked at the amount of noise that was going on around him and Eleanor. He realised that the suggestion that she might not be able to hear him could indeed be true. He was also surprised that he had not noticed how loud the everyday environment was, or if he had when he first started working at Roseford, then he had obviously got used to it.

Once they were in the quiet room James positioned Eleanor's wheelchair and brought a chair so that he was sitting at the side of her facing her. He looked at Eleanor and spoke her name while also gently rubbing her arm. She moved slightly and looked down at his hand touching her arm. 'How are you?' he asked her as he stroked her arm again. She looked up into his eyes then down again at her arm. She screwed her face up a bit and then relaxed it and looked quickly at James. She then looked back at her arm and kept her gaze there for three or four seconds before turning her head slightly away from James.

James reached out his hand to touch her again and she turned her head back and looked at his hand on her arm. He moved his hand and she turned her head away again. James then asked, 'Did you enjoy your breakfast, Eleanor?' and she turned to look quickly at him again. She kept his gaze for a couple of seconds then turned away and then straight back. It looked like head shaking and James asked 'Was that a 'No?' Eleanor looked down at James' hand and then closed her eyes. While her eyes were closed, her mouth started moving in a sort of chewing motion. James tried to copy this movement but Eleanor's eyes were closed so she did not see him. She then turned her head away from James and opened her eyes and looked down at her other hand. She moved her head slowly and looked at her arm nearest to James, which she then started moving. She also moved her mouth again as her fingers moved.

James asked her if she was tired and Eleanor looked straight into his eyes and made more mouth movements. She alternately looked at James, looked at her hand nearest to him, and closed her eyes. She then turned her head away and James stroked her arm and she wrinkled her nose. She slowly turned back to him and looked at him and then her arm. She kept her gaze down on her arm and his nearby hand then lifted her head slowly to look at James again. This time she held his gaze and James was delighted and surprised. He felt that he had made a connection and he couldn't wait to share the experience with Betty and Stacey and the rest of the group.

Fundamentals of Communication	
1. Eye gaze	Eleanor started with her eyes closed. When I touched her arm she looked down at my hand. She then looked at my face and for the rest of the session she looked at me, down at her arm, looked away or closed her eyes.
2. Facial expressions	I would say that Eleanor's facial expression was mostly neutral but she did wrinkle up her nose a couple of times when I touched her.
3. Speech/speech sounds	There was no speech at all from Eleanor.
4. Sounds	She didn't make any sound.
5. Physical contact	I stroked her arm several times.
6. Gestures	She turned her head away from me a few times and she also moved her arm that was nearest to me.
7. Imitation	I'm not sure if there was imitation until the end when she was looking right at me and I was looking at her.
8. Bodily position	She was sitting up in her wheelchair facing me.
9. Emotion	She did not seem to like me touching her as she frowned or wrinkled her nose. She seemed to be paying attention to me.
10. Turn-taking	We did take turns this time! It was really clear to me when I was reflecting the movement of her mouth and when she reacted to me touching her arm or speaking to her.

Chart 6.4 Connecting with Eleanor

We can see from Chart 6.4 above that James is beginning to think differently about how he might connect with Eleanor and what that might look like. Although she did not seem to like him touching her arm – she screwed up her face or wrinkled her nose – whenever he did it, she looked at her arm and his hand. He noticed that her gaze kept moving from her arm, to his hand, his face or body as well as turning away. But she always turned back and finally they were gazing at each other. He was both proud and excited as he felt they had made a connection. He now had a way to reach Eleanor and he could use this next time he saw her. However, the AI trainer reminded him that what 'works' one day might not do so the next. Even though he knew what had happened, there was no way of knowing if Eleanor would also remember and so he had to approach each interaction afresh. However, he could do this knowing that he had made a connection once and that he should aim to do this every time. Keeping this in mind, James looked forward to his next interaction with Eleanor, all the while wondering what might happen next.

Step 5: Building the connection

The final session of the AI training was looming and James wanted to put in plenty of practice with Eleanor before it was done. He knew the trainees would continue to use the approach with their communication partners and he wanted to have a role in taking the approach forward at Roseford Care Home. The following passage describes the last session between Eleanor and James during the training period.

This time James made sure that Eleanor was sitting upright before he started the session. He had asked a colleague to help him to get her comfortable in a padded chair in her room. She was quiet when he entered. He said hello and drew up a chair beside her when she could see him. He sat down in his chair, smiled at Eleanor and gently touched her arm with his little finger. As he did so he said 'hello' and she immediately frowned and moved her arm away (Chart 6.5). They sat for a few seconds and then Eleanor moved her arm slightly back towards James. He moved his hand and very gently stroked her arm again. She lifted her arm to her body and looked down at his hand. Eleanor began moving her mouth in the way she had before and James started to gently tap on the arm of her chair in concert with the rhythm. Eleanor watched James' hand intently and he realised he could hear her breathing as she looked at his hand moving. She started to move her head a little and shifted her eyes between his hand and her lap. Gradually she started moving her fingers and James changed his hand movement to match Eleanor's. After several seconds, she lifted her arm again and put it back across her chest.

Eleanor then moved her hand to her lap and began pinching at the material of her skirt, effectively starting a new phase of the interaction. James responded immediately by making the same movements at the other side just above but not directly on her skirt. Eleanor would look at her hand, then James', backwards and forwards for several minutes. Just briefly and only a few times, she glanced up and made eye contact with James. She kept alternating her gaze between his hand and hers and, briefly, his face. He moved his hand to stroke her arm and this time she moved slightly away but then back again. He carried on gently stroking and she kept her arm there and started moving her fingers.

This continued for about a minute and then Eleanor lifted her arm but immediately put it back. Her fingers and her mouth were moving as James continued to gently stroke her arm. She lifted her arm away and made more mouth movements. James did the same and kept his gaze firmly on her face. After about 30 seconds she slowly lifted her hand and placed it on top of James'. Eleanor eventually ended the interaction by closing her eyes and stopping her hand movements. When he was sure she was safely asleep, James left Eleanor's room. He was grinning from ear to ear.

Fundamentals of Communication	
1. Eye gaze	Eleanor looked backwards and forwards at her own hands then at mine. She briefly made eye contact with me a few times but mainly she looked at my hand or her hand or had her eyes closed.
2. Facial expressions	Eleanor's facial expression was mostly neutral. She frowned initially when I touched her arm but did not do this later in the session.
3. Speech/speech sounds	No speech – don't think this category is relevant for Eleanor.
4. Sounds	I realised I could hear her breathing when I was stroking her arm.
5. Physical contact	I gently stroked her arm and she kept it there for longer and longer periods. Finally, she lifted her arm and put her hand on mine.
6. Gestures	Eleanor pushed my hand away when I touched her arm at the beginning of the interaction. I'm still learning!

7. Imitation	I saw lots of imitation this time. Sometimes I would follow what she was doing with her hand and sometimes she followed me.
8. Bodily position	I made sure that Eleanor was sitting upright in a chair before we started the session as this seems to be the position in which she is most alert.
9. Emotion	She may have been unhappy when I first touched her arm but later she seemed contented when I stroked her and she was moving her fingers.
10. Turn-taking	We took lots of turns this time. Lots of to and fro with hand movements.

Chart 6.5 Building the connection with Eleanor

Group discussion

James was looking forward to telling everyone about his latest interaction with Eleanor and was excited to go into the final feedback session. There was much discussion among the trainees about what they had discovered, both about themselves and their communication partners. James was feeling proud of himself and of Eleanor. They had really achieved something together.

What follows is James' part of the discussion.

Trainer: James – how would you say you have got on with the training?

James: I felt like I was making a really rotten job of it to begin with.

Trainer: Oh no! Why is that?

James: I really didn't think I had the knack and I felt that the others were way ahead of me in terms of what they had managed to achieve with their communication partners. As you know, I'm quite new to this job and I worry a lot that I might be getting all sorts of things wrong!

Trainer: So, what's changed for you?

James: Well, I managed to find a way of interacting with Eleanor that seemed pleasant for her. To begin with, I felt like she really didn't want to engage with me at all. However, I found that if I kept my distance at the start she would let me get closer to her. She just needed a bit of time to get used to it, especially physical contact.

Trainer: Fantastic! It says a lot about you that you were willing to carry on. At what point did you feel you had made a breakthrough?

James: I saw a difference in Eleanor when I concentrated on where she was looking and alternating that with moving my hand. She really seemed to pay attention to my hand and then she looked up and met my eyes. It felt amazing to have 'met' her, if you like.

Trainer: And were you able to take that forward?

James: Yes, I was able to spend more time with her and I realised I did not need to rush to get a response. However, sometimes when I went to see her she didn't respond to the things I tried. I guess on those occasions I wasn't focusing on what she was doing and instead was thinking about what had 'worked' for her before.

Trainer: Absolutely. I believe that Eleanor actually reached out and touched your hand – is that right?

James: Ha! Yes – she did! I was completely flabbergasted! I've always been told that she hates being touched and that that's why she gets so upset during personal care.

Trainer: So, do you think that using Adaptive Interaction could make a difference to how she responds to personal care?

James: I think we could try a few things with her and see how we get on. Using touch has to be on her terms so it might be that we interact with her using her language for a while before we start personal care.

Trainer: It's interesting that you say that. Shouldn't we be using her language to communicate with her *all* the time?

James: Yes, of course. Practice makes perfect!

Trainer: Exactly! What do you think is the most important lesson you have learned over the course of the training?

James: I think realising that communication is possible without speech is the first thing. When I watch Eleanor and Mike eating chocolates and holding hands together, I see more than I did before. It holds more meaning for me. Second, I see my job as something more than I did before this training. I feel more confident in myself now. I'm someone who is valuable and who brings joy to people. That's an amazing thing to be able to say.

Summary

Eleanor's story has shown us that – as if we didn't know already – we should not judge a book by its cover. Sounds obvious, doesn't it? However, we form opinions of other people not just by our own experiences with them but also via conversations with others. The interactions that occurred between James and Eleanor suggest that she is more afraid than hostile and that a little perseverance goes a long way. Mike and Angie are delighted with how James and Eleanor have connected and they really hope this will pave the way for changes in how all the staff care for and interact with Eleanor.

Chapter 7

The Sound of Silence

Bert's Story

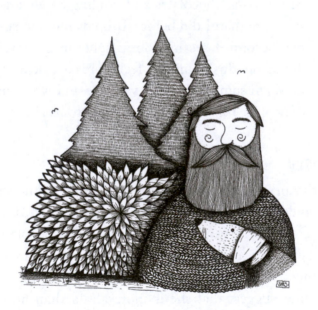

This chapter tells more of Bert's story. We learn about his background and his current communication repertoire. This chapter describes in detail how we might communicate with someone with advanced dementia who is extremely quiet and seemingly non-communicative.

Bert

Bert is 85 years old and has been living in Roseford Care Home for the past five years. He is a very quiet and gentle man who spent his working life as a ranger at a local wildlife park. He retired at 65 and enjoyed a peaceful and relatively solitary existence until he was 79 years old. Before moving to Roseford, Bert was somewhat of a loner and spent most of his time walking in the woods with his dog, Isla. Although outwardly friendly, he had no close friends or family and never married or had a partner. Bert's passion in life was nature and as such the outdoor life of a park ranger suited him. He tended to avoid large groups, preferring instead to keep himself to himself.

Bert was diagnosed with dementia when he was 79 years old. His neighbours became concerned when he started walking Isla in the middle of the night. Sometimes the dog would return home on her own and Bert would spend the night looking for her. One night, Bert's neighbour Betty found Isla, still in her collar and lead, barking outside her companion's door at 4 a.m. She took the dog indoors and her husband Frank went out to look for Bert. Frank found Bert in the woods near his home. He was physically well but very confused, cold and upset. That evening's events prompted Betty and Frank to keep an eye on Bert thereafter. They would visit him every day and he would bring Isla over to their house on Sundays for dinner. Bert seemed to enjoy their company despite his retiring nature and always looked genuinely pleased to see them. It seemed to Betty and Frank that all Bert needed was someone to make the first move and show an interest in him.

Bert changed significantly over the course of the following year. Betty and Frank noticed that he was losing weight and becoming unsteady on his feet. Frank started to walk Isla to help out and sometimes Bert would forget who his neighbour was when he came to the door. Eventually Bert refused to open the door to his neighbours and they would hear Isla barking and howling in distress. Frank and Betty called social services as they were so concerned about Bert and Isla's welfare. He was assessed and quickly moved to Roseford as he was deemed no longer able to care for himself or for his dog. Betty and Frank adopted Isla and still take her to visit him at the care home to this day.

Bert is now confined to his bed as he can no longer walk. He doesn't talk now and seems to be completely unaware that he has company when Frank, Betty and Isla come to visit. He doesn't make eye contact and never utters a sound. He mostly spends his days sleeping and when he *is* awake, he seems to stare into space. Frank and Betty find it very upsetting to see Bert like this and visit him less and less these days. Bert has almost no opportunities for social interaction outside the visits from his neighbours and dog, as some of the staff at Roseford do not feel he is able to communicate.

Let's now think about what life might be like for Bert and how he might be feeling when he awakes from sleep. Since he is unlikely to remember where he is, try to imagine that Bert may have a similar experience each time he wakes up.

BERT'S PERSPECTIVE

Bert is asleep. He dreams of a walk in the woods, the smell of the clean air and the sound of running water. He hears the songs of the birds, the wind in the trees and the panting of his dog and her paws plodding along the path behind him. Bert is in his 'happy place' – the place where he feels most at home, most alive. Although it is a wild environment, Bert feels as though he is in control. He knows this woodland path like the back of his hand. He knows every tree, every bench and every rambler. This is his domain and one that he loves. All of a sudden, he can feel his eyelids flutter and he sees a bright light overhead. Bert is awake – but where? He feels a huge shock to his senses as he looks around this very strange-looking room. He is lying down and tries to move but can't. His arms are trapped underneath a blanket. He tries to call for help but finds he can produce no more than a faint moan. Bert is frightened and confused. He has no idea where he is and there is no-one nearby he can look to for help.

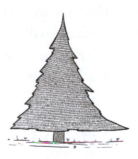

How, then, does Bert feel about his life and surroundings? How can we tell if he doesn't speak or seem to communicate in any way at all? The truth of the matter is that we can't expect to be able to understand what Bert is thinking in any sort of concrete way. He no longer seems to be able to produce speech or understand what is said to him. As such, we do not even know if his thoughts are based in speech any more. When humans think, we tend to do so in words, although we may not be consciously aware of this. For example, around 12 noon you might feel your stomach rumble, which signals to you that you are 'hungry'. You might then start thinking to yourself about what you might have for lunch – 'Should I choose the healthy option and have a baked potato or should I get something I really fancy, like macaroni cheese?' Although we can never know for certain, we *can* assume to some extent that Bert doesn't have the full capacity to think in words or to form mental sentences. Because we are so used to communicating using speech, it becomes extremely difficult for us to imagine what it must be like to live without it. As such, for us to consider what Bert is thinking becomes almost impossible.

Perhaps now it becomes possible to consider communicating with Bert in another way. Could we maybe consider what he is *feeling* rather than what he is thinking? This may be a simpler, more intuitive way to connect with Bert, in that tapping into 'happy', 'sad' or 'bored' might be easier for us to understand than trying to decipher his thoughts. This is a difficult concept to get your head around at first but thinking back to the example in Chapter 2 of going to the cinema will help. Can you imagine now how Bert might feel when he awakes? He is likely to experience uncertainty, fear, helplessness and isolation. Why?

He may feel:

- **uncertain** because he has no idea where he is or who the people are who surround him

- **afraid** because he is completely disorientated and the world he inhabits doesn't make sense to him

- **helpless** because he can't participate in the world around him

- **isolated** because he cannot form thoughts or words to express himself.

Betty

Betty is 65 years old and was Bert's neighbour for ten years before he was diagnosed with dementia. A couple of her friends have relatives with dementia but she has never been close to anyone with a diagnosis before she became friends with Bert. She knew Bert as an active, quiet but friendly man and finds it very difficult to see him as he is now. She likes Roseford and appreciates everything that the staff do for her friend. However, she feels that he is lost to her and lonely.

Let's now look a little more closely at Bert's situation from Betty's perspective.

BETTY'S PERSPECTIVE

Betty and Frank came to visit Bert at Roseford this morning. They brought Isla, Bert's dog, with them as they thought he might like to see her. When they entered the room, Bert was asleep. He was facing the wall and didn't stir when they came in. Betty sighed when she saw Bert. She hated to see him like this – a man who was always on the go, now confined to bed. She and Frank walked towards Bert's bed. Isla sniffed Bert and wagged her tail in recognition but Bert didn't stir. Frank gently tapped Bert's shoulder to let him know he had visitors. Bert immediately rolled over on his back and opened his eyes. Betty and Frank smiled and said hello but Bert still didn't respond. They tried a few more times to engage him by telling him the local gossip and about the walks they had been on with Isla. However, they soon gave up. Bert didn't look at them and didn't seem to be listening to them either. He stared somewhere into the middle distance and appeared to be in his own world.

This was a common pattern to their visits, which Betty came to dread. He was just so different from the man she remembered. He had always been a quiet, unassuming man but it seemed he had nothing left at all now. He didn't look at her or Frank, he didn't make a sound and, perhaps most surprising of all, he didn't seem to recognise or to want to interact with Isla. She had been his constant companion and Betty felt as though he had completely cut himself off from his pet too. None of it made sense to Betty. She knew bits and pieces about dementia and how it can affect people but she had never seen anyone affected like this before. Like Bert, she felt uncertainty, fear, helplessness and isolation.

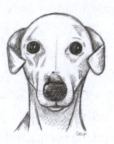

You may be surprised to learn that Bert and Betty are likely to experience similar emotions in response to the situation they find themselves in. Although Betty is aware of what has happened to Bert, of where he is and why he is there, she experiences similar feelings to him but for different reasons.

- She feels **uncertain** because she doesn't know if Bert can hear her or if he is aware that she is there.

- She feels **afraid** in that she doesn't want to approach Bert in case he doesn't respond to her.

- She experiences **helplessness** because she feels that she just can't get through to Bert and that there is no way of doing so.

- She also experiences a sense of **isolation** because she feels cut off from Bert and that he is unwilling to communicate with her.

Without even knowing it, Betty and Bert are already connected in terms of the similarities in feelings they are likely to be experiencing. One of the main aims of AI is to address these feelings for both people with dementia and their caregivers and to strive to achieve the opposite feelings. For example, if we believe that Bert might be feeling uncertainty, then we should strive to make him feel certainty. If we think he feels fear, then we should help him to feel unafraid. If he seems to be helpless, then we should try to help him to feel in control. If he seems to be experiencing isolation then we should strive to include him. The same goes for Betty. If we strive to change our own feelings in response to working with individuals with dementia then we not only improve our own wellbeing, we also experience feelings of empowerment and the pride of having achieved something wonderful.

What is clear from Betty's perspective is that we can only experience these types of realisations if we are willing to consider that communication might be possible without speech. We can see that Bert doesn't seem to respond to conversation but that we witness some sort of response via an alternative path (touch). Maybe we need to travel a different route to reach him – to meet him there. As we saw in Chapter 4, the process of assessing and using a person's communication repertoire involves some trial and error to find out what 'works'. And what works for one person will not necessarily do so for another. This means that we are required to be committed to finding a way of connecting to each person and that we regard every individual as just that – an individual. However, there will undoubtedly be obstacles along the way – usually in the form of other people. The idea of a person using an alternative form of communication is not an easy one to comprehend. As the developers of AI, we have most certainly met with disbelief in terms of what is possible in the work that we do. However, this soon melts away as people see the results and feel the level of connection that occurs when we communicate with people with dementia using AI.

So, it seems we have two individuals – one with additional communication needs and one typical communicator – who can't reach each other. Betty would love to be able to interact with Bert but he doesn't seem interested or able to do so. But how can we know for sure that Bert is unwilling and unable to communicate? It certainly looks to be the case as he doesn't respond when Betty talks to him. He is completely silent. However, if we look a little deeper we can see something that Bert *did* respond to. When Frank tapped him on the shoulder to let him know his friend was there, Bert rolled over. Could it be that Bert 'understands' touch? Betty experienced a lightbulb moment – perhaps she could use touch as a way in to Bert's world. What Betty doesn't realise at this point is that she is already thinking about using AI to communicate with Bert. This needn't be that surprising, as this type of 'alternative' communication is one that occurs quite naturally in other situations. As you read in Chapter 1, we typically interact with very young infants in this way – using the communicative actions that they produce to interact with them. We also communicate with peers in a similar way. You may have in-jokes with a particular friend that would be meaningless to another of your close companions. This is a form of language that you have co-created and is a way in which you have collaborated to develop understanding. You may even have a look that you use to communicate something with a friend or partner and you both know what each other is 'talking about'.

PAUSE FOR THOUGHT: THE PARTY

You and your best friend are at a school reunion. Neither of you *really* wanted to go but you conclude that it might be fun to meet up with some old friends and to see what everyone is up to these days. The reunion is held in a hotel ballroom and there are lots of people milling about so you take care to stay close together. Suddenly you feel a tap on your shoulder and you turn around to find your first boyfriend standing there smiling at you. Instead of asking you how you are and starting an exchange, he launches into what seems like a well-rehearsed script of his achievements and successes over the last 25 years! His job, wife, kids, house – everything sounds so perfect and it's clear that he's trying to impress you. This continues for what seems like an age and you turn to your friend widening your eyes and raising your eyebrows, ever so slightly. Your friend then looks over your shoulder and waves over to the far side of the ballroom. She squeezes your hand and says, 'Oh look – it's Carol waving us over! We haven't seen her in years!' You look at your ex and say, 'Sorry – it looks like I have to go and see Carol! It was nice talking to you – 'bye for now!'

If the above situation sounds familiar to you it's because it's the sort of unspoken code that occurs between close friends and partners all the time. It seems intuitive and simple but when you break it down into its component parts it's actually quite a complex interaction. The look you gave your friend communicated several different pieces of information. No words were exchanged between you but she could tell that:

- you weren't enjoying the interaction with your ex

- you wanted her to help you to get out of the situation

- it had to be subtle enough so that your ex-boyfriend wouldn't be offended.

This goes to show that even the smallest gesture can tell us so much about how someone is feeling.

Training in Adaptive Interaction

Betty has heard that the staff at Roseford are about to start a training programme in AI. The manager thought that training in the approach would benefit staff, residents and family members in that it would provide a means of connection. Betty wondered if she might be able to take part in the training as she had heard so much about it and it sounded like something that might allow her to get through to Bert in some way. The manager agreed and Betty attended the first session. She was a little nervous about taking part in something she thought was designed for professional caregivers but she felt excited to be part of it.

On the first day of the training programme, participants were taught about AI and where the approach originates from. You, of course, will have read all about this in the first few chapters of this book. There were certain parts of the first training session that Betty found a little uncomfortable. For example, hearing that AI grew from developmental theory (how infants develop) made her wonder how appropriate this approach would be for adults. She reasoned that although people with dementia like Bert have severe communication difficulties, they are not babies and are not the same as babies. Betty raised this point with the trainer and the other trainees nodded in agreement. The trainer fully agreed with Betty and explained that the fundamental communication skills that are utilised in AI are not specific to infants – we all use them. The trainer went on to explain that these skills are intrinsically human in nature and, as such, they occur across the lifespan. The trainees soon got the hang of this idea using some of the examples you have already read in this book. Before the training began, the participants were partnered with a person with advanced dementia whom they already knew. Of course, Betty was paired with Bert.

Step 1: Getting to know Bert

As we saw in Chapter 4, the first stage of the AI process is to assess how much information you know about the person you will be working with. The chart below (Chart 7.1) was completed by Betty about Bert. She was in a favourable position in that she knows lots about him and knew him well before he became ill.

You will notice that the last two categories of the chart require Betty to write down how she thinks Bert might be feeling and how she herself is feeling. As we saw earlier, this is important to note, as with AI we attempt to reverse these feelings.

Getting to Know You	
How much personal information do you know about the person, e.g. previous occupation, number of children, hobbies?	Bert's full name is Robert Gordon Walker. He was a park ranger before he took ill and loved the outdoors. He never married or had any children. He loves animals, the countryside and being active.
What do you know about the person's life before he/she became ill?	Bert lived with his dog, Isla, before he became ill. He had two main friends – his neighbours, Frank and Betty (me!).
What are the person's likes and dislikes?	Bert doesn't like to be the centre of attention. He prefers the quiet life and likes to spend a lot of time alone. He does like to have company sometimes but it has to be on his own terms. He loves animals (especially dogs), nature and being outdoors.
What are the obstacles to communicating with this person?	Bert is extremely silent these days and I haven't heard him make a sound in all the times I have visited him. He doesn't make eye contact either and it's very difficult to know whether or not he is hearing or understanding me or, indeed, whether or not he is aware that anyone is there.
How do you think he might be currently feeling and why?	I think he might be feeling uncertain because he has no idea where he is or who the people are who surround him. He may also be afraid because he seems completely disorientated. Bert may also be feeling helpless because he can't participate in anything. I believe that he may also be feeling isolated because he doesn't seem able to communicate with us.
How do you feel when you try to interact with him and why?	I feel uncertain because I don't know if Bert can hear me or if he is aware that I'm there. I'm apprehensive because I don't want to approach Bert in case he doesn't respond to me. I often feel helpless because I just can't get through to Bert and I feel that I never will. I feel isolated and cut off from Bert because he seems to be either unwilling or unable to communicate with me.

Chart 7.1 Getting to Know Bert

Although at first glance, the information that Betty provided about Bert doesn't seem to amount to much, we will find later that some of this information is vital in finding a way to interact with him.

Step 2: The communication environment

The second part of the training, as described in Chapter 4, involves analysing the 'communication environment'. Betty felt a little strange about taking notes on what she saw happening in Bert's environment – she didn't want the staff to think she was spying on them. However, Betty had explained this part of the process to those who weren't taking part in the training this time and there were no complaints. Chart 7.2 gives Betty's summary of what she saw in Bert's communication environment.

The Communication Environment	
How often does someone interact with this person in a typical day?	I would say a maximum of four staff members interacted with Bert over the last two days. Apart from meal times and being helped to the toilet, etc. he is left pretty much to himself. I have been here a lot over the past two days as I'm doing the training and have been chatting away to Bert as usual.
What 'type' of communication most often occurs? 'Functional' (task-based) or 'social'?	Most of the communication I have seen with the staff is task-based and happens when there is a 'job' to be done. I try to engage in social interaction with Bert but I feel as though I'm talking to myself as I never seem to get a reaction from him.

Chart 7.2 Bert's Communication Environment

Step 3: Identifying the communication repertoire

As we saw in Chapter 4, the next step of the AI process involves identifying the individual communicative repertoires of each person with dementia. This is done via entering interactions with the communication partner and using the Fundamentals of Communication chart to reflect on the communication. All of the interactions that trainees and their communication partners engage in together during the training period are video recorded by another trainee. This allows the trainees and trainers to analyse what has happened during the interactions and to see them in more detail. Betty and the other trainees feel apprehensive about being videoed but the trainer assures them that this is an essential element of the programme and that they will soon get used to being filmed and may even forget that the camera is there!

The first part of this process is to engage in a five-minute 'typical' interaction with the person with dementia to whom you are partnered. What we mean by this is that you would interact with the person as you normally would, which could mean different things for different people. Betty went to Bert's room and sat by his bed. She was apprehensive about approaching him even though she had spoken to him perhaps hundreds of times over the years. The reason she felt uneasy is that she wasn't sure exactly how she *normally* went about interacting with Bert. She thought back to the times she had visited him over the last few weeks and she realised that she largely spoke to him – but why? He didn't respond to her and she could never tell whether or not he could hear or understand her. Therefore, in order to 'do' something with Bert she brought with her a yoghurt and some milk that she would help him to eat and drink.

Bert was asleep when Betty entered his room. She approached him slowly and quietly so as not to startle him. The cot-sides of Bert's bed were up so Betty had to lean over him to interact. She said hello to Bert and he opened his eyes but didn't look directly at her. She told him she had a drink and a yoghurt for him and told him she would to prop him up a bit so he could have them. Bert's jaw was moving from side to side almost as though he was eating already. As Betty moved towards him to plump his pillows he opened his mouth wide in expectation. 'Two seconds', said Betty, then she put the spout of the beaker to his lips. Bert drank with great fervour for a few swallows, then broke off. He started rolling his tongue around in his mouth and Betty asked him if he would like some more. She put the spout to his lips and he had another few sips. This pattern repeated several more times until the milk was finished. Some of the milk was running down Bert's chin and Betty told him she was going to give it a wipe. Just as she was getting a cloth, Bert started to rub the side of his head and face. Betty thought he must have an itch, and wiped the milk from his lips. Bert screwed up his face a little – it seemed he didn't like having his chin wiped! Betty asked Bert if he was hungry and she took his hand. He immediately responded by wrapping his fingers around hers. Betty was surprised – Bert had never tried to hold her hand before! Feeling encouraged, Betty continued to get Bert's yoghurt ready. She put the spoon to his lips and he opened his mouth. Bert never made eye contact or any sounds with Betty while she was helping him to eat. However, she was used to him being this way and felt that despite this, Bert had a level of understanding of what was going on. Bert looked up at the ceiling and Betty asked him what he could see. He continued to look up and finished his yoghurt.

Betty's interaction with Bert highlights three main points. First, Betty felt too uncomfortable to go and sit with Bert without having something to 'do', so she brought food and drink with her to give her something to focus on. Second, the interaction served to confirm Betty's feeling that Bert didn't really respond to speech in any way that she could easily identify. Third, and most surprising to Betty, Bert seemed to respond to touch. When she took his hand, he grasped it and she realised she hadn't felt that close to him since before he came to live at Roseford. She thought that this might be a way in to reach Bert again. Betty's Fundamentals of Communication chart for the interaction just described is shown in Chart 7.3.

Fundamentals of Communication	
1. Eye gaze	Bert looked either past me or up to the ceiling throughout the interaction. He didn't make eye contact with me and I couldn't figure out what, if anything, he was looking at.
2. Facial expressions	Sometimes it was hard to tell what Bert's facial expressions were or might be as he was eating and drinking during the session. However, if I had to guess I would say he maintained a neutral expression throughout.

3. Speech/speech sounds	Bert didn't produce any speech.
4. Sounds	He didn't make any sounds at all.
5. Physical contact	I took Bert's hand at one point and he grasped my hand in return. I was quite shocked by this and pleasantly surprised!
6. Gestures	The only gestures I could see were Bert opening his mouth in anticipation of his food and drink. However, this does seem to suggest a level of understanding of what was happening around him.
7. Imitation	I couldn't see Bert imitate anything I was doing.
8. Bodily position	Bert was lying flat on his back when I entered the room.
9. Emotion	I struggled to see any sort of emotional response from Bert.
10. Turn-taking	I couldn't identify any turn-taking either.

Chart 7.3 Bert's communication repertoire

Looking at Betty's chart we can see that she has struggled to identify communicative actions in Bert. She didn't think that there was very much going on between them until Bert grasped her hand. This is the starting point for Betty and Bert. She has noted that touch might be a good way of connecting with Bert and is encouraged by the rest of the trainees and the trainer to give it a try. However, this also sparked a lively discussion when they watched the video together. James voiced his concern about using touch with his communication partner as it might be misconstrued by those around her. A few of the other trainees nodded in agreement, with one stating that she would feel uncomfortable using touch to communicate with a member of the opposite sex. The trainer thanked the trainees for making these extremely valid points, explaining that she had heard this argument many times over the years. She asked the group to remember that we follow the lead of the person with dementia in AI. If he is using touch as a means of connecting with you then you can try using it with him in return. As long as you use your common sense and are comfortable with it, touch can be a wonderful way of connecting with someone. Betty was heartened by this advice and was excited to try the next interaction with Bert.

Step 4: Creating a connection

Betty was eager to move on to step 4 of the Adaptive Interaction process. She was fascinated by the idea that she might be able to connect with Bert by using touch. Like the rest of the trainees, she felt a little nervous as it's not something she had ever considered before. She had known Bert to be very shy and reserved and she found it surprising to find that something as intimate as touch could provide them with a means of interacting. However, she had definitely witnessed a response and was willing to give it a try.

Betty entered Bert's room. The first thing she noticed was that the staff member who had been in the room before her had left the radio on. It was tuning in and out and it crackled. Betty told Bert she was going to switch it off as it was a 'racket'. She then walked over to his bed and leaned in closer to him than she had the last time. She wished him good morning and took his hand in hers. To her surprise he gripped her hand and started to squeeze it rhythmically and quite quickly. She responded immediately by doing the same with her hand. She noticed that Bert's jaw was moving as it had been the other day but it was much faster this time. Then, all of a sudden, Bert looked at Betty. She was elated! He wasn't one for making eye contact and she felt she had somehow made a breakthrough with him. They continued to hold and squeeze each other's hands and Betty told Bert she had a yoghurt for him and asked, 'Are you hungry?' Bert let go of Betty's hand and moved his hand up the side of his head and over the top, then rubbed the back of his head. Betty asked him if his head was itchy but he didn't look at her. Bert put his hand back down on the bed and Betty gently stroked his forearm, asking him again if he was hungry. He then started rubbing the back of his head again. Betty broke away from Bert and went to fetch his yoghurt. Bert was still rubbing the side of his face and over to the back of his head when Betty asked, 'Are you ready for your yoghurt?' Bert lay still. Betty told Bert that it was strawberry today and put the spoon to his lips. Bert held Betty's gaze while she fed him his yoghurt. She spoke to him softly and gently about Frank coming to visit with Isla and about Isla being fed treats by the staff.

When Bert finished his yoghurt, he looked up to the ceiling. Betty noticed a new mobile hanging there and asked Bert if someone had made it for him. Bert stayed silent but continued to watch the mobile move above his head. He started rubbing the side of his face around to the back of his head again and Betty took this cue to replicate the rhythm of this on Bert's forearm. The two continued like this for the remainder of the session. Bert would occasionally make eye contact with Betty which made her feel as though she was really getting somewhere with him. Chart 7.4 shows Betty's Fundamentals of Communication chart for the interaction just described.

Fundamentals of Communication	
1. Eye gaze	Bert made eye contact with me on several occasions. This felt really special as I haven't seen him do this in such a long time. He also looked up to the ceiling at his new mobile from time to time.
2. Facial expressions	I think Bert mostly had a neutral facial expression but it was sometimes hard to tell as he was eating and moving his jaw around a lot.
3. Speech/speech sounds	No speech.
4. Sounds	Bert didn't make any sounds.
5. Physical contact	There was much more physical contact between us than there was last time. I took Bert's hand and he squeezed it in almost a rhythmic way. When Bert was moving his hand up the side of his face and over his head, I tried to replicate the rhythm of it on his forearm.
6. Gestures	Several times Bert would rub the side of his face and move his hand up and over the top of his head. He would do this repeatedly, always in the same order. He also moved his jaw from side to side quite a lot this time. Like last time, Bert also opened his mouth in anticipation of food.

7. Imitation	I didn't identify any imitation.
8. Bodily position	Like last time, Bert was lying flat on his back except when I raised the bed so he could eat.
9. Emotion	I still didn't see an emotional response from Bert.
10. Turn-taking	Again, I couldn't identify any turn-taking.

Chart 7.4 Connecting with Bert

The above chart illustrates Betty and Bert's progress together. Betty still didn't feel confident enough to go into Bert's room empty-handed. She brought a yoghurt with her and helped him to eat it, giving her something to do if the interaction didn't go as well as she imagined it might. Nevertheless, it's clear that Betty was becoming more confident. We can see this in her actions and descriptions of her getting physically closer to Bert, in her recognising 'new' communicative behaviours in him and in her own broadening range of responses. We can also see that Bert is now making eye contact with Betty – something that is unusual for him to say the least. He is also holding and squeezing her hand. Just to be clear, this doesn't necessarily mean that Bert is developing new communicative behaviours. Rather, it is much more likely that Betty is recognising and responding more to him, thereby eliciting a wider range of his existing communicative repertoire.

Step 5: Building the connection

Betty has learnt a lot over the course of the Adaptive Interaction training programme and feels closer to Bert than she has in years. In fact, she feels even *closer* to Bert than before as she is starting to develop the skills to interact with him without the need to talk. Yes, she is still using speech now and again but not as much as before and she is beginning to feel more and more confident about using touch to communicate with him. It is through this mode of communication that Bert is best able to respond and Betty feels she needs to work on this more to get even closer to him. What follows is a description of one of Betty and Bert's last interactions within the training period.

The first thing Betty did during this session was to move the cot-side of Bert's bed down as far as it could go. That way she could get in as close to him as he was comfortable with. She then sat down beside Bert but slightly in front of him so he could see her as well as possible. Bert's right hand was on top of the blankets at his side and his left was clenched at the side of his neck. Bert made eye contact with Betty straight away and she took his right hand. He squeezed her hand and looked directly into her eyes. Bert was rolling his tongue around in his mouth and it looked as though he was making speech-like shapes with his lips. Betty was face to face with Bert and began lightly tapping his left hand, reflecting the rhythm he made with his mouth. They carried on like this for a while and Bert would move his and Betty's clasped hands around in the air from time to time. Betty eventually let go of Bert's hand and he began moving his fingers in a scrabbling and scratching movement on the side of the bed. Betty did the same with her hand at his other side, then tapped out the corresponding rhythm very lightly on Bert's chest. Bert didn't take his eyes off Betty at all and it felt both intense and relaxing to Betty – a slightly strange but wonderful combination. They were connecting. Betty stroked Bert's clenched left hand and he moved his hand up the side of his face and over the top of his head. This definitely seemed to be one of Bert's signature communicative actions. Bert then brought his hand back down onto the blankets and began scratching the covers again. Betty tried to repeat the rhythm on the covers and Bert's fingers moved closer and closer to her. After a while, Betty felt confident enough to try something new – she tried stroking the side of Bert's face and up and over his head as he does. When she did this, Bert looked surprised at first but then his face lit up with the faintest of smiles. Betty couldn't be sure of what she was seeing and returned to Bert's right hand to reflect his scratching movement. She placed her hand on top of his, using little strokes to imitate his movement, then she moved her hand away. Bert then quickly moved his hand towards Betty's and reached out for hers. This was amazing! Bert had never reached out for Betty before – she felt this really was a breakthrough! Encouraged by this, Betty stroked Bert's face and head again and there it was – a huge smile! They smiled at each other for what felt like an age and Betty came back to the group feeling like she had really achieved something amazing. Chart 7.5 shows Betty's Fundamentals of Communication chart for this interaction.

Fundamentals of Communication	
1. Eye gaze	Bert made constant eye contact with me throughout this session. It felt wonderful and not at all awkward – which I guess is strange in itself!
2. Facial expressions	Other than a largely neutral expression, Bert definitely smiled a couple of times during this interaction. This was amazing as I haven't seen him smile in years!
3. Speech/speech sounds	Bert didn't use any words.
4. Sounds	He didn't make any sounds.
5. Physical contact	There was lots of physical contact during this session. Bert reached out for my hand which was lovely! I also stroked his face and head – I think that was what made him smile!
6. Gestures	Bert made scratching movements with his fingers and rubbed the side of his face and up and over his head. He also moved his hand to hold mine.
7. Imitation	I did see imitation this time. When we were 'scratching' on the blankets, I moved my hand in one direction and Bert followed.
8. Bodily positio	Again, Bert was lying on his back but I was much closer to him than in previous sessions.
9. Emotion	I think I can safely say that Bert was happy – I saw him smile! He was also very engaged and interactive.
10. Turn-taking	There was definitely some turn-taking going on this time. The 'scratching' of our fingers felt like a game – you do this, then I do the same.

Chart 7.5 Building the connection with Bert

Group discussion

Betty was eager to tell the trainer and other trainees about her interaction with Bert at the final group discussion of the training. She also wanted to discuss how she might take things further and to keep things going after the training ended. What follows is Betty's part in the discussion.

Trainer: Hello Betty, you're looking pretty happy! How do you feel the training has gone?

Betty: I think it's gone much better than I thought it ever could and I have managed to reconnect with my friend. It's really a lovely feeling!

Trainer: Oh, that's wonderful! Can you tell us how you think you achieved that?

Betty: I'll try! – I think the training in Adaptive Interaction had afforded me a deeper understanding of what communication actually is. That it's not just about talking about what we watched on the telly last night or what we think of Mrs so-and-so's new hairdo. I now look for things that I wouldn't have previously considered to be of any value.

Trainer: Good. Can you elaborate?

Betty: Yes, I think so. I began the training by always bringing something with me – a prop almost. I would bring Bert something to eat or drink mostly because I was worried that I would run out of things to do. I was worried I would feel awkward or even helpless. When I look back at the early sessions, it's only now that I realised how much I talked!

Trainer: Why do you think you did that?

Betty: Because that's just how you communicate normally, isn't it? It's like a safety blanket of sorts. You learn how to fill awkward silences and to make social situations feel a little more comfortable by talking. That in itself is a kind of prop, isn't it? Because I am now more aware that Bert doesn't speak and probably doesn't understand what other people are saying to him, I have to find his level – to meet him where he is if you like.

Trainer: That's a great way of putting it! What do you think you will try next with Bert now that the training is finished?

Betty: I know this might sound silly but I'd like to bring Bert's dog Isla in when I interact with him. They were inseparable in the past and he doesn't seem to recognise her now. Also, animals were always a big part of his life and I think finding a way of reintroducing her to him might be of great benefit to Bert. To Isla too, come to think of it!

Trainer: I don't think that sounds silly at all! They already communicated in the past without speech so they're halfway there! How do you think you will go about doing that?

Betty: Now that I know that touch is so significant to Bert, I think the first thing I'll try will be to help him to pet Isla. Perhaps take his hand and move it over her so that he can feel her fur again.

Trainer: That sounds like a great idea. I'd be really interested to hear how you get on with that.

Summary

Bert's story has shown us that despite him being a quiet and reserved man, he still needs human connection. Probably more now than ever, Bert needs to know and to feel that he is part of something, part of a social world: a world where he matters and is important to other people. Perhaps now, carers will be more likely to visit Bert in his room just to interact with him. They might try taking him to the day room more often or encourage him to sit with other residents. Betty hopes that one day Bert will be able to interact with his dog, Isla, and perhaps get some pleasure from seeing her. Helping Bert to touch and stroke Isla might help – then again, it might not. What we want for those we care for doesn't always happen. We don't always get to have the fairy-tale ending. Following our communication partner's lead is always the way forward in AI and we can't make 'meaning' for the person. We make meaning *together*.

Epilogue

So, now you have read this book we hope you feel excited about AI and can envisage the benefits that it will bring to you and those you love and care for. While eliciting the desire to interact with individuals with dementia is certainly one of the main aims of this book, we hasten to add that it is not designed to be a 'how to'. Rather, this book serves as an introduction to AI and to the theory and research that underpins it. Effective use of the approach at home or in care facilities requires careful planning, a sound knowledge base and closely supervised practice and feedback. This is provided via validated training programmes and we have a range of these to help both individuals and organisations to start using AI safely and ethically. Please visit us at www.astellis.co.uk for further information.

We thank you for your interest in AI and sincerely hope that you find it as exciting and gratifying as we do. We'd like to finish with a few quotes from some of our trainees.

> 'The main thing I learned was that nonverbal communication is far more beneficial to a lot of our clients than trying to communicate verbally because a lot of them are further on in their dementia.'

'It makes you think a bit more when you're communicating – I find it calms clients down when they are agitated.'

'We take communication for granted and even though some of the residents can't communicate verbally we assume that they understand us. When we use Adaptive Interaction we can see that they pay more attention and the focus is on you and them.'

'It's rewarding when you see you're getting somewhere. It's beneficial for ourselves and the clients.'

'I found that Adaptive Interaction brought something out of the clients that was hidden. Even if it was only blinking an eye, it was blinking an eye in response to something that we had done. Before, we wouldn't recognise it but with the training we realised that it was a response to us. Using this technique, I felt that I got something back and that it made my job easier. That blink of an eye means something, that movement of the hand means something.'

'The family members saw something in their loved ones that they hadn't seen for many years.'

'Taking a step back and watching the residents' body language – I couldn't believe the difference it made.'

'This should be something that is done regularly. It needs to be a part of training like everything else.'

'Even family members saw a difference and that's probably the hardest thing.'

Appendix

Adaptive Interaction Process Charts

The assessment form templates from this appendix
are available to download and print from
www.jkp.com/catalogue/book/9781785921971

Getting to Know You chart

Getting to Know You
How much personal information do you know about the person, e.g. previous occupation, number of children, hobbies?
What do you know about the person's life before he/she became ill?
What are the person's likes and dislikes?
What are the obstacles to communicating with this person?
How do you think he/she might be currently feeling and why?
How do you feel when you try to interact with him/her and why?

Communication Environment chart

The Communication Environment
How often does someone interact with this person in a typical day?
What 'type' of communication most often occurs? 'Functional' (task-based) or 'social'?

Fundamentals of Communication chart

Communicators' names:	Date:	Time:

Fundamentals of Communication
1. Eye gaze
2. Facial expressions
3. Speech/speech sounds
4. Sounds
5. Physical contact

6. Gestures

7. Imitation

8. Bodily position

9. Emotion

10. Turn-taking

References

Almberg, B., Grafström, M. and Winblad, B. (1997). Major strain and coping strategies as reported by family members who care for aged demented relatives. *Journal of Advanced Nursing, 26* (4), 683–691.

Alzheimer, A. (1907). A characteristic disease of the cerebral cortex. In K. Bick, L. Amaducci and P. Giancarlo (eds), *The Early Story of Alzheimer's Disease.* Padova, Italy: Liviana Press.

Alzheimer's Disease International (2015). Dementia Friends. www.alz.co.uk/dementia-friendly-communities/dementia-friends (accessed 5 April 2017).

Astell, A. J. and Ellis, M. P. (2006). The social function of imitation in severe dementia. *Infant and Child Development, 15*(3), 311–319.

Astell, A. J., Ellis, M.P., Alm, N., Dye, R. and Gowans, G. (2010). Stimulating people with dementia to reminisce using personal and generic photographs. *International Journal of Computers in Healthcare, 1*(2), 177–198.

Astell, A. J., Ellis, M. P., Bernardi, L., Bowes, M., Tunnard, C. and Webb, H. (2005). *A Review of the Needs of People with Dementia and Their Caregivers.* Unpublished review prepared for CRAM International Ltd, London, UK.

Astell, A. J., Ellis, M. P. and Hockey, H. J. (2004). Social cognition in dementia. *Journal of Cognitive Neuroscience,* supplement, 126.

Aström, S., Nilsson, M., Norberg, A., Sandman, P. O. and Winblad, B. (1991). Staff burnout in dementia care – relations to empathy and attitudes. *International Journal of Nursing Studies, 28*(1), 65–75.

Azuma, T. and Bayles, K. (1997). Memory impairments underlying language difficulties in dementia. *Topics in Language Disorders, 18*(1), 58–71.

Baker, R., Angus, D., Conway, E., Baker, K. S., Gallois, C., Smith, A., et al. (2015). Visualising conversations between care home staff and residents with dementia. *Ageing and Society First View, 35*(2), 1–28.

Batty, M. and Taylor, M. J. (2003). Early processing of the six basic facial emotional expressions. *Cognitive Brain Research, 17*(3), 613–620.

Bayles, K. A. and Tomoeda, C. K. (1991). Caregiver report of prevalence and appearance order of linguistic symptoms in Alzheimer's patients. *Gerontologist, 31*(2), 210–216.

Bayles, K. A. and Tomoeda, C. K. (1993). *Arizona Battery for Communication Disorders of Dementia*. Austin, TX: PRO-ED.

Beach, S. R., Schulz, R., Williamson, G., Miller, L. S., Weiner, M. F. and Lance, C. E. (2005). Risk factors for potentially harmful informal caregiver behaviour. *Journal of the American Gerontological Society, 53*, 255–261.

Berg, A., Hansson, U. W. and Hallberg, I. R. (1994). Nurses' creativity, tedium and burnout during 1 year of clinical supervision and implementation of individually planned nursing care: comparisons between a ward for severely demented patients and a similar control ward. *Journal of Advanced Nursing, 20*(4), 742–749.

Bird, M., Llewellyn-Jones, R., Smithers, H. and Korten, A. (2002). Psychosocial approaches to challenging behaviour in dementia: a controlled trial. Canberra: Department of Health and Ageing.

Bowie, P. and Mountain, G. (1993). Using direct observation to record the behaviour of long stay patients with dementia. *International Journal of Geriatric Psychiatry 8*, 857–864.

Brooker, D. (2003). What is person-centred care in dementia? *Reviews in Clinical Gerontology, 13*(3), 215–222.

Brooker, D. (2006). *Person-Centred Dementia Care: Making Services Better*. London: Jessica Kingsley Publishers.

Buber, M. (1958). *I and Thou*, translated by Ronald Gregor Smith. New York: Scribners.

Bull, P. (2002). *Communication Under the Microscope: The Theory and Practice of Microanalysis*. Hove, UK: Routledge.

Burgio, L. D., Engel, B. T., Hawkins, A., McCormick, K. and Scheve, A. (1990). A descriptive analysis of nursing staff behaviors in a teaching nursing home: differences among NAs, LPNs, and RNs. *Gerontologist, 30*(1), 107–112.

Burgoon, J. K., Buller, D. B., Hale, J. L. and de Turcke, M. A. (1984). Relational messages associated with nonverbal behaviours. *Human Communication Research, 10*(3), 351–378.

Burgoon, J. K., Guerrero, L. K. and Floyd, K. (2009) *Nonverbal Communication*. Boston, MA: Allyn and Bacon.

Caldwell, P. (2005). *Finding You Finding Me: Using Intensive Interaction to Get in Touch with People whose Severe Learning Disabilities Are Combined with Autistic Spectrum Disorder*. London: Jessica Kingsley Publishers.

Caldwell, P. (2008). Intensive Interaction; Getting in Touch with a Child with Severe Autism. In S. Zeedyk (ed.) *Techniques for Promoting Social Engagement in Individuals with Communicative Impairments*. London: Jessica Kingsley Publishers.

Caldwell, P., Hoghton, M. and Mytton, P. (2010). *Autism and Intensive Interaction: Using Body Language to Reach Children on the Autistic Spectrum*. London: Jessica Kingsley Publishers.

Caldwell, P. and Horwood, J. (2007). *From Isolation to Intimacy: Making Friends without Words*. London: Jessica Kingsley Publishers.

Campbell, N. (2007). On the Use of Nonverbal Speech Sounds in Human Communication. In A. Esposito, M. Faundez-Zanuy, E. Keller & M. Marinaro (eds) *Verbal and Nonverbal Communication Behaviours*, Lecture Notes in Computer Science 4775. Berlin: Springer.

Carstensen, L.L., Fisher, J.E. and Malloy, P.M. (1995). Cognitive and affective characteristics of socially withdrawn nursing home residents. *Journal of Clinical Geropsychology, 1*(3), 207–218.

Chappell, N. L. and Novak, M. (1992). The role of support in alleviating stress among nursing assistants. *Gerontologist, 32*(3), 351–359.

Chatterjee, A., Strauss, M. E., Smyth, K. A. and Whitehouse, P. J. (1992). Personality changes in Alzheimer's disease. *Archives of Neurology, 49*(5), 486–491.

Clark, H. H. and Brennan, S. E. (1991). Grounding in communication. In L. B. Resnick, J. M. Levine & S. D. Teasley (eds.) *Perspectives on Socially Shared Cognition*. Washington, DC: APA.

Clark, H. H. and Wilkes-Gibbs, D. (1986). Referring as collaborative process. *Cognition, 22*, 1–39.

Coia, P. and Jardine Handley, A. (2008). Developing relationships with people with profound learning disabilities through intensive interactions. In M. S. Zeedyk (ed.) *Promoting Social Interaction for Individuals with Communicative Impairments*. London: Jessica Kingsley Publishers.

Constable, J. F. and Russell, D. W. (1986). The effect of social support and the work environment upon burnout among nurses. *Journal of Human Stress, Spring*(1291), 20–26.

Darwin, C. (1872). *The Expression of Emotion in Man and Animals*. New York: Oxford University Press.

Day, J. R. and Anderson, R. A. (2011). Compassion fatigue: an application of the concept to informal caregivers of family members with dementia. *Nursing Research and Practice*, doi: 10.1155/2011/408024.

Dijkstra, K., Bourgeois, M., Petrie, G., Burgio, L. and Allen-Burge, R. (2002). My recaller is on vacation: discourse analysis of nursing-home residents with dementia. *Discourse Processes, 33*(1), 53–76.

Duffy, M. (1999). Reaching the person behind the dementia. In M. Duffy (ed.) *Handbook of Counselling and Psychotherapy in Older Adults*. New York: Wiley.

Ellis, M. P. and Astell, A. J. (2004). The urge to communicate in severe dementia. *Brain and Language, 91*(1), 51–52.

Ellis, M. P. and Astell, A. J. (2008). Promoting Communication with People with Severe Dementia. In S. Zeedyk (ed.) *Techniques for Promoting Social Engagement in Individuals with Communicative Impairments*. London: Jessica Kingsley Publishers.

Ellis, M.P. and Astell, A. J. (2017). Communicating with people living with dementia who are nonverbal: The creation of Adaptive Interaction. *PLoS One, 12*(8), e0180395.

Ernst, P. and Shaw, J. (1980). Touching is not taboo. *Geriatric Nursing, 1*(3), 193–195.

Feast, A., Orrell, M., Charlesworth, G., Melunsky, N., Poland, F. and Moniz-Cook, E. (2016). Behavioural and psychological symptoms in dementia and the challenges for family carers: systematic review. *British Journal of Psychiatry, 208*(5), 429–434.

Feil, N. (1993). *The Validation Breakthrough: Simple Techniques for Communicating with People with Alzheimer's-Type Dementia*. Baltimore, MD: Health Professions Press.

Feldman, R., Singer, M. and Zagoory, O. (2010). Touch attenuates infants' physiological reactivity to stress. *Developmental Science, 13*, 271–278.

Galati, D., Miceli, R. and Sini, B. (2001). Judging and coding facial expressions in congenitally blind children. *International Journal of Behavioral Development, 25*(3), 268–278.

Gleeson, M. and Timmins, F. (2004). Touch: a fundamental aspect of communication with older people with dementia. *Nursing Older People, 16*(2), 18–21.

Goldin-Meadow, S., Mylander, C. and Franklin, A. (2007). How children make language out of gesture: morphological structure in gesture systems developed by American and Chinese deaf children. *Cognitive Psychology, 55*(2), 87–135.

Gratier, M., Devouche, E., Guellai, B., Infanti, R., Yilmaz, E. and Parlato-Oliveira, E. (2015). Early development of turn-taking in vocal interacitons between mothers and infants. *Frontiers in Psychology, 6*, 1167.

Gutmanis, I., Snyder, M., Harvey, D., Hillier, L. M. and LeClair, J. K. (2015). Health care redesign for responsive behaviours—the Behavioural Supports Ontario experience: lessons learned and keys to success. *Canadian Journal of Community Mental Health, 34*(1), 45–63.

Haden, C. A. (1998). Reminiscence with different children: relating maternal stylistic consistency and sibling similarity in talk about the past. *Developmental Psychology, 34*, 99–114.

Harlow, H. (1958). The nature of love. *American Psychologist, 13*, 673–685.

Hartling, L. M. and Luccheta, T. (1999). Humiliation: assessing the impact of derision, degredation, and debasement. *Journal of Primary Prevention, 19*(4), 259–278.

Hazelhof, T.J.G.M., Schoonhoven, L., van Gaal, B. G. I., Koopmans, R.T.C.M. and Gerritsen, D. L. (2016). Nursing staff stress from challenging behaviour of residents with dementia: a concept analysis. *International Nursing Review, 63*(3), 507–516.

Hepburn, K. W., Tornatore, J., Center, B. and Ostwald, S. W. (2001). Dementia family caregiver training: affecting beliefs about caregiving and caregiver outcomes. *Journal of the American Geriatrics Association, 49*(4), 450–457.

Hershman Shitrit, M. and Cohen, J. (2016). Why do we enjoy reality shows: is it really all about humiliation and gloating? *Journal of Media Psychology*, doi: 10.1027/1864-1105/a000186.

Hertenstein, M. J., Verkamp, J. M., Kerestes, A. M. and Holmes, R. M. (2006). The communicative functions of touch in humans, nonhuman primates, and rats: a reviews and synthesis of empirical research. *Genetics Society General Psychology Monograph, 132*, 5–94.

Hewett, D. (1996) How to Do Intensive Interaction. In M. Collis and P. Lacey (eds) *Interactive Approaches to Teaching: A Framework for INSET*. London: David Fulton.

Ho, S., Foulsham, T. and Kingstone, A. (2015). Speaking and listening with the eyes: gaze signaling during dyadic interactions, *PLOS ONE, 10*(8), e0136905.

Hobson, P. (1993). *Autism and the Development of Mind*. Hillsdale, NJ: Lawrence Erlbaum Assoc.

Holler, J., Hendrick, K. H., Casillas, M. and Levinson, S. C. (2015). Editorial: Turn-taking in human communicative interaction. *Frontiers in Psychology, 6*, 1919.

Holt-Lunstad, J., Birmingham, W. C. and Light, K. C. (2014). Relationship quality and oxytocin influence of stable and modifiable aspects of relationships. *Journal of Social and Personal Relationships, 32*(4), 472–490.

Iacoboni, M. (2009). Imitation, empathy, and mirror neurons. *Annual Review of Psychology, 60*, 653–670.

International Telecommunication Union (ITU) (2015). ITU releases 2015 ICT figures. www.itu.int/net/pressoffice/press_releases/2015/17.aspx#.WT0pFMaZNPs

Iverson, J. and Goldin-Meadow, S., (1997). What's communication got to do with it? Gesture in children blind from birth. *Developmental Psychology, 33*(3), 453–467.

Katzman, R. (1976). The prevalence and malignancy of Alzheimer's disease. *Archives of Neurology, 33*(4), 217–218.

Katzman, R. and Karasu, T. B. (1975). Differential Diagnosis of Dementia. In W. Fields (ed) *Neurological and Sensory Disorders in the Elderly*. New York: Grune and Stratton.

Kellett, M. (2000). Sam's story: evaluating Intensive Interaction in terms of effect on the social and communicative ability of a young child with advanced learning difficulties. *Support for Learning, 15*(4), 165–171.

Kellett, M. (2003). Jacob's journey: developing sociability and communication in a young boy with severe and complex learning difficulties using the intensive interaction teaching approach. *Journal of Research in Special Educational Needs, 3*(1), 116–121.

Kitwood, T. (1990). The dialectics of dementia: with particular reference to Alzheimer's disease. *Ageing and Society, 10*(2), 177–196.

Kitwood, T. (1997). *Dementia Reconsidered: The Person Comes First*. Buckingham: Open University Press.

Kitwood, T. and Bredin, K. (1992). Towards a theory of dementia care: personhood and well-being. *Ageing and Society, 12*(3), 269–287.

Kleinke, C. L. (1986). Gaze and eye contact: a research review. *Psychological Bulletin, 100*(1), 78–100.

Knapp, M. L. and Hall, J. A. (2010). *Nonverbal Communication in Human Interaction*, 7th edition. Wadsworth, Canada: Cengage Learning.

Koder, D., Hunt, G. E. and Davison, T. (2014). Staff's views on managing symptoms of dementia in nursing home residents. *Nursing and People, 26*(10), 31–36.

Krauss, R. M. (2005). The Psychology of Verbal Communication. In N. Smelser & P. Baltes (eds) *International Encyclopedia of the Social and Behavioral Sciences*. London: Elsevier.

Lhommet, M. and Marsella, S. C. (2015). Expressing Emotion through Posture and Gesture. In R. Calvo, S. D'Mello, J. Gratch & A. Kappas (eds) *The Oxford Handbook of Affective Computing, Oxford Library of Psychology*. Oxford: Oxford University Press.

Lima, E. D. R. S. and Cruz-Santos, A. (2012). Aquisição dos gestos na comunicação pré-linguística: uma abordagem teórica Acquisition of gestures in prelinguistic communication: a theoretical approach. *Rev Soc Bras Fonoaudiol, 17*(4), 495–501.

Lubinski, R. (1995). State of the art perspectives on communication in nursing homes. *Topics in Language Disorders, 15*(2), 1–19.

MacDonald, G. and Leary, M. R. (2005). Why does social exclusion hurt? The relationship between social and physical pain. *Psychological Bulletin, 131*(2), 202–223.

Mast, J. (2016). The dark side of reality TV: professional ethics and the treatment of reality show participants. *International Journal of Communication, 10,* 2179–2200.

Matsumoto, D. and Hwang, H. S. (2011). Reading facial expressions of emotion. Psychological Science Agenda, Science Brief. Washington, DC: APA. www.apa.org/science/about/psa/2011/05/facial-expressions.aspx (accessed 4 July 2017).

Medina, J. and Weintraub, S. (2007). Depression in primary progressive aphasia. *Journal of Geriatric Psychiatry and Neurology, 20*(3), 153–160.

Mehrabian, A. (1971). *Silent Messages.* Belmont, CA: Wadsworth Publishing.

Meltzoff, A. N. and Moore, M. K. (1983). Newborn infants imitate adult facial gestures. *Child Development, 54*(3), 702–709.

Moniz-Cook, E., Woods, B. and Gardiner, E. (2000). Staff factors associated with perception of behaviour as 'challenging' in residential and nursing homes. *Ageing and Mental Health, 4*(1), 48–55.

Nadel, J., Croué, S., Mattlinger, M-J., Canet, P., Hudelot, C., Lécuyer, C., et al. (2000). Do children with autism have expectancies about the social behaviour of unfamiliar people? A pilot study using the still face paradigm. *Autism, 4*(2), 133–145.

Neal, M. and Barton Wright, P. (2003). Validation therapy for dementia. *Cochrane Database of Systematic Reviews, doi:* 10.1002/14651858.CD001394.

Nelson, K. (1985). *Making Sense: The Acquisition of Shared Meaning.* New York: Academic Press.

Newson, J. (1978). Dialogue and Development. In A. Lock (ed.) *Action, Gesture and Symbol: The Emergence of Language.* New York: Academic Press.

Nind, M. (1996). Efficacy of Intensive Interaction: developing sociability and communication in people with severe and complex learning difficulties using an approach based on caregiver–infant interaction. *European Journal of Special Educational Needs, 11*(1), 48–66.

Nind, M. (1999). Intensive Interaction and autism: a useful approach? *British Journal of Special Education, 26*(2), 96–102.

Nind, M. and Hewett, D. (1994) *Access to Communication: Developing the Basics of Communication with People with Severe Learning Difficulties through Intensive Interaction.* London: David Fulton.

O'Donnell, B. F., Drachman, D. A., Barnes, H. J., Peterson, K. E., Swearer, J. M. and Lew, R. A. (1992) Incontinence and troublesome behaviors predict institutionalization in dementia. *Journal of Geriatric Psychiatry and Neurology, 5*(1), 45–52.

Ong, D. C., Goodman, D. C. and Zaki, J. (2017). Happier than thou? A self-enhancement bias in emotion attribution. *Emotion,* doi: 10.1037/emo0000309.

Onyike, C. U. and Diehl-Schmid, J. (2013). The epidemiology of frontotemporal dementia. *International Review of Psychiatry, 25*(2), 130–137.

Orange, J. B., Lubinksi, R. B. and Higginbotham, D. J. (1996). Conversational repair by individuals with dementia of the Alzheimer's type. *Journal of Speech and Hearing Research, 39*(4), 881–895.

Orange, J. B. and Purves, B. (1996). Conversational discourse and cognitive impairment: implications for Alzheimer's disease. *Canadian Journal of Speech–Language Pathology and Audiology, 20*(2), 151–153.

Orange, J. B., Ryan, E. B., Meredith, S. and MacLean, M. J. (1995). Application of the communication enhancement model for long-term residents with Alzheimer's disease. *Topics in Language Disorders, 15*(2), 20–35.

Oxford Dictionaries (2015). Oxford Dictionaries Word of the Year. http://blog. oxforddictionaries.com/2015/11/word-of-the-year-2015-emoji (accessed 5 April 2017).

Oxford English Dictionary (2011). March 2011 update: New initialisms in the OED. http://public.oed.com/the-oed-today/recent-updates-to-the-oed/previous-updates/march-2011-update (accessed 5 April 2017).

Papoušek, M. (1995). Origins of reciprocity and mutuality in prelinguistic parent–infant 'dialogues'. In I. Markova, C. F. Graumann, & K. Foppa (eds) *Mutualities in Dialogue*. Cambridge: Cambridge University Press.

Paton, J., Johnston, K., Katona, C. and Livingston, G. (2004). What causes problems in Alzheimer's disease: attributions by caregivers. A qualitative study. *International Journal of Geriatric Psychiatry, 19*(6), 527–532.

Perrin, T. (2001). Don't despise the fluffy bunny: a reflection from practice. *British Journal of Occupational Therapy, 64*(3), 129–134.

Prince, M., Wimo, A., Guerchet, M., Gemma-Claire, A., Wu, Y-T. and Prina, M. (2015). *World Alzheimer Report 2015. The Global Impact of Dementia: An Analysis of Prevalence Incidence, Cost and Trends*. London: Alzheimer's Disease International. www.alz.co.uk/research/WorldAlzheimerReport2015.pdf (accessed 4 July 2017).

Quinn, C., Clare, L. and Woods, B. (2009). The impact of the quality of relationship on the experiences and wellbeing of caregivers of people with dementia: a systematic review. *Ageing and Mental Health, 13*, 143–154.

Raia, P. (1999). Habilitation Therapy: A New Starscape. In L. Volicer (ed.) *Enhancing the Quality of Life in Advanced Dementia*. New York: Brunner/Mazel Publishers.

Raia, P. (2011). Habilitation therapy in dementia care. *Age in Action, 26*(4), 2–6.

Raia, P. and Koenig-Coste, J. (1996). Habilitation therapy. *Alzheimer's Association of Eastern Massachusetts Newsletter, 14*(2), 1–2, 4–6.

Rayner, K., Bradley, S., Johnson, G., Mrozik, J. H., Appiah, A. and Nagra, M. K. (2014). Teaching intensive interaction to paid carers: using the 'communities of practice'model to inform training. *British Journal of Learning Disabilities*, doi: 10.1111/bld.12111.

Ripich, D. N. (1994). Functional communication with AD patients: a caregiver training program. *Alzheimer's Disease and Associated Disorders, 8* (Supplement 3), 95–109.

Robinson, L., Clare, L. and Evans, K. (2005). Making sense of dementia and adjusting to loss: psychological reactions to a diagnosis of dementia in couples. *Ageing and Mental Health, 9*(4), 337–347.

Rommetveit, R. (1974). *On Message Structure: A Framework for the Study of Language and Communication*. New York: Wiley.

Samuel, J. and Maggs, J. (1998). Introducing Intensive Interaction for People with Profound Learning Disabilities Living in Small Staffed Houses in the Community. In D. Hewett, and M. Nind (eds) *Interaction in Action: Reflections on the Use of Intensive Interaction*. London: David Fulton Publishers.

Savundranayagam, M. Y., Sibalija, J. and Scotchmer, E. (2016). Resident reactions to person-centred communication by long-term care staff. *American Journal of Alzheimer's Disease and Other Disorders, 31*(6), 530–537.

Seligman, M. E. P. (1972). Learned helplessness. *Annual Review of Medicine, 23*(1), 407–412.

Shea, S. C. (1998). *Psychiatric Interviewing: The Art of Understanding*, 2nd edition. Philadelphia, PA: Sanders.

Shenk, D. (2001). *The Forgettng: Alzheimer's: Portrait of an Epidemic*. New York: Anchor.

Simmons, S. F., Durkin, D. W., Rahman, A. N., Choi, L., Beuscher, L. and Schnelle, J. F. (2013). Resident characteristics related to the lack of morning care provision in long-term care. *Gerontologist, 53*(1), 151–161.

Smith, M. and Buckwalter, E. (2005). Behaviors associated with dementia: whether resisting care or exhibiting apathy, an older adult with dementia is attempting communication. Nurses and other caregivers must learn to hear this language. *American Journal of Nursing, 105*(7), 40–52.

Springate, B. A. and Tremont, G. (2014). Dimensions of caregiver burden in dementia: impact of demographic, mood and care recipient variables. *American Journal of Geriatric Psychiatry, 22*(3), 294–300.

Stivers, T., Enfield, N. J., Brown, P., Englert, C., Hayashi, M., Heinemann, T., et al. (2009). Universals and cultural variation in turn-taking in conversation. *Proceedings of the National Academy of Sciences*, doi: 10.1073/pnas.0903616106.

Stokes, G. (2000). *Challenging Behaviour in Dementia. A Person-Centred Approach*. Milton Keynes: Speechmark Publishing Ltd.

Stoppe, G., Brandt, C. and Staedt, J. (1999). Behavioral problems associated with dementia. The role of newer antipsychotics. *Drugs and Aging, 14*, 41–54.

Swaffer, K. (2013). Talking, dementia and humiliation [Blog post]. https://kateswaffer.com/2013/01/22/talking-dementia-and-humiliation (accessed 4 July 2017).

Sweeting, H. and Gilhooly, M. (1997). Dementia and the phenomenon of social death. *Sociology of Health and Illness, 19*(1), 93–117.

Tennakoon, K. L. U. S. and Taras, D. G. (2012). The relationship between cell phone use and sense of security: a two-nation study. *Security Journal, 25*(4), 291–308.

Tomasello, M. (1992). The social bases of language acquisition. *Social Development, 1*(1), 67–87.

Trevarthen, C. (2004). Learning about Ourselves, from Children: Why a Growing Human Brain Needs Interesting Companions. *Research and Clinical Center for Child Development Annual Report, 26*, 9–44.

Valenza, E., Simion, F., Macchi-Cassia, V. and Umiltà, C. (1996). Face preference at birth. *Journal of Experimental Psychology: Human Perception and Performance, 22*, 892–903.

Vygotsky, L. S. (1978). *Mind in Society: The Development of Higher Psychological Processes*. Cambridge, MA: Harvard University Press.

Wiersma, E. C. and Denton, A. (2016). From social network to safety net: dementia-friendly communities in rural northern Ontario. *Dementia, 15*(1), 51–68.

Woods, R. T. (1999). Psychological Therapies in Dementia. In R. T. Woods (ed.) *Psychological Problems of Ageing*. Chichester: Wiley.

Woods, R. T., Keady, J. and Seddon, D. (2007). *Involving Families in Care Homes: A Relationship-Centred Approach to Dementia Care*. London: Jessica Kingsley Publishers.

Zarit, S. H. and Edwards, A. B. (2008). Family Caregiving: Research and Clinical Interventions. In R. T. Woods & L. Clare (eds) *Handbook of the Clinical Psychology of Ageing*, 2nd edition. New York: John Wiley & Sons, Ltd.

Zephoria Digital Marketing (2017). The Top 20 Valuable Facebook Statistics – Updated July 2017. https://zephoria.com/top-15-valuable-facebook-statistics (accessed 9 July 2017).

Subject Index

Sub-headings in *italics* indicate charts and figures.

Author Index